Yoga & DIABETES

D0572474

YOUR GUIDE
TO SAFE AND
EFFECTIVE
PRACTICE

ANNIE B. KAY, MS, RDN, RYT and Lisa B. Nelson, MD

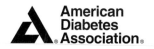

**American
Diabetes
Association.**

Director, Book Publishing, Abe Ogden; Managing Editor, Greg Guthrie; Acquisitions Editor, Victor Van Beuren; Project Manager, Kim Douglass Marin; Production Manager, Melissa Sprott; Cover Design and Composition, pixiedesign, llc; Photographer, Gregory Cherin Photography; Printer, RR Donnelley.

Printed in the United States of America

1 3 5 7 9 10 8 6 4 2

The suggestions and information contained in this publication are generally consistent with the *Standards of Medical Care in Diabetes* and other policies of the American Diabetes Association, but they do not represent the policy or position of the Association or any of its boards or committees. Reasonable steps have been taken to ensure the accuracy of the information presented. However, the American Diabetes Association cannot ensure the safety or efficacy of any product or service described in this publication. Individuals are advised to consult a physician or other appropriate health care professional before undertaking any diet or exercise program or taking any medication referred to in this publication. Professionals must use and apply their own professional judgment, experience, and training and should not rely solely on the information contained in this publication before prescribing any diet, exercise, or medication. The American Diabetes Association—its officers, directors, employees, volunteers, and members—assumes no responsibility or liability for personal or other injury, loss, or damage that may result from the suggestions or information in this publication.

Maria Mupanomunda, MD, PhD, MBA, conducted the internal review of this book to ensure that it meets American Diabetes Association guidelines.

♾ The paper in this publication meets the requirements of the ANSI Standard Z39.48-1992 (permanence of paper).

ADA titles may be purchased for business or promotional use or for special sales. To purchase more than 50 copies of this book at a discount, or for custom editions of this book with your logo, contact the American Diabetes Association at the address below or at booksales@diabetes.org.

American Diabetes Association
1701 North Beauregard Street
Alexandria, Virginia 22311

DOI: 10.2337/9781580405577

Library of Congress Cataloging-in-Publication Data
Kay, Annie
 Yoga and diabetes : your guide to safe and effective practice / Annie B. Kay and Lisa B. Nelson, MD.
  pages cm
 Includes bibliographical references and index.
 ISBN 978-1-58040-557-7 (spiral bound)
 1. Diabetes--Exercise therapy. 2. Yoga--Therapeutic use. I. Nelson, Lisa. Title.
 RC661.E94N45 2015
 616.4'62062--dc23
        2014042715

To my yoga teachers, including Barbara Benagh in
Boston, Bhavani Maki in Kauai, my Nantucket Yoga
Room colleagues, and so many others; and to my yoga
teacher/colleagues at Kripalu, who have done no less
than help me tend the best of myself. Deep bows of
gratitude for my lineage and what you have shown me.
ANNIE

To Stephen, Madeleine, and Hannah,
for your support, encouragement, and patience.
LISA

Contents

Acknowledgments

Like most worthwhile book projects, this one is the work of many hands and minds.

Many thanks to our colleagues at the Kripalu Center for Yoga & Health in Stockbridge, Massachusetts, for being friendly to our "round peg" project. Thanks to David Lipsius and Stephen Daoust for your support and for taking a certain leap of faith, and to Ellen Rose Cunningham, Silvia Eggenberger, and Eric Hoffman for organizing and taking care of us.

The photo shoot for this project was hosted by and held on the beautiful grounds of Kripalu, which is the largest yoga-based retreat center in North America.

Thanks to Laurie Magoon for assistance in a pinch, Janna Delgado for your sweet classiness, and Mark Natale for stepping in with a serving heart. You were perfect! Thanks to Greg Cherin for the gorgeous photography. Monique Richard, thank you for your review of the yoga postures included in the book.

Thanks to the American Diabetes Association publishing team of Victor Van Beuren, Greg Guthrie, Kim Marin, and Katie Curran, and the scientific review panel for making this yoga offering possible.

In gratitude,
Annie B. Kay, MS, RDN, RYT
Lisa B. Nelson, MD

Foreword

Yoga has become very popular in the U.S., with a 2012 national survey revealing that fully 9% of the population is actively practicing these ancient techniques. Furthermore, the fact that the percentage of practitioners in similar surveys in 2002 and 2007 was 5% and 6%, respectively, suggests that this popularity is growing very rapidly.

Many of these practitioners are benefitting from yoga's positive influence on stress management, emotion regulation, mind-body awareness/mindfulness, and physical fitness. It is likely that the increase in stress in modern society, together with the lack of behavioral life skills available in our medical and education systems for managing stress and enhancing mind-body awareness, has fueled this attraction for yoga practices.

Furthermore, yoga has become popular as a therapeutic intervention, either as health and wellness maintenance and illness prevention, or as an adjunct or even primary therapy to treat an existing medical or psychological condition. Scientific research is confirming the physical and psychological improvements that can be achieved with yoga practice, and a growing body of clinical research trials is demonstrating that yoga practices have efficacy in a wide variety of clinical disorders. A number of research studies have demonstrated that yoga is useful for disorders of glucose regulation, whether in the form of prediabetes, metabolic syndrome, or type 2 diabetes.

Improvements have been demonstrated in measures of blood glucose, mood, stress, and quality of life, and a few studies have shown positive improvements at the cellular and biochemical level with respect to insulin and glucose regulation. It is probably not a coincidence that the growing level of yoga practice and research on its efficacy is coming at a critical time in the nation's health.

The greatest burden in our current health-care system is clearly the large and increasing prevalence of so-called non-communicable diseases. These disorders, which include obesity, depression, cardiovascular disease, and type 2 diabetes, are the greatest contributor to mortality and health-care costs, are at near-epidemic proportions, and are significantly growing in prevalence. These are diseases largely driven by poor lifestyle choices and behaviors, which are in turn due in part to an inability to cope with stress and to a lack of mind-body awareness. Sedentary behavior, poor dietary choices, and chronic unmanaged stress are key factors contributing to lifestyle diseases.

Unfortunately, our modern medical system has a strong emphasis on symptom treatment and disease management, and it has largely focused on technological or pharmaceutical treatment approaches. It has not been as strong as it needs to be on primary prevention and on addressing the underlying behavioral causes for these lifestyle disorders.

Yoga practice has a significant potential for addressing key lifestyle and behavioral issues with disorders such as type 2 diabetes. Research supports the significant role of yoga practices in reducing stress and enhancing resilience and emotion regulation, which are of key importance in diabetic or metabolic syndrome patients. Yoga research studies have also shown improvements in mind-body awareness and mindfulness. These are important factors in that they encourage adoption of positive lifestyle behaviors because of patients' improved experience of the benefits of healthy activities. Patients will choose increased physical activity because they enjoy experiencing the positive physical changes. They will engage in less stress-induced overeating, be more in tune with their inherent satiety during meals, and be more aware of the effects of positive food choices.

Yoga therefore has significant potential as a bottom-up approach to lifestyle change in patients and is likely to support their success in complying with their health-care providers' recommendations for healthy lifestyle behaviors. A strong argument can be made for the need for inclusion of mind-body practices such as yoga into both the education and health-care systems, with their potential to prevent the growing epidemic in lifestyle disease in modern society.

Sat Bir Singh Khalsa, PhD

Assistant Professor of Medicine, Brigham and Women's Hospital, Harvard Medical School
Director of Research, Kundalini Research Institute
Research Associate, Benson-Henry Institute for Mind Body Medicine
Director of Research, Kripalu Institute for Extraordinary Living

Preface

In my lifetime, yoga has blossomed from an esoteric oddity to a mainstream fashion trend. It seems everyone is "doing" yoga, and stores from Sears to Neiman Marcus carry mats and yoga clothes. The variety of yoga styles is as endless as the American imagination—truly boundless! If you are so moved, you can now take up hula-hoop yoga, acrobatic circus yoga, or take a yoga and meditation vacation at a monastery. According to Yoga Journal magazine's most recent survey, more than 20 million Americans practice yoga, and that number continues to grow.

What is all the fuss about? Part of the interest is our natural curiosity about things that are new, different, and from far away, and yoga certainly is that. But much of yoga's popularity is due to its unique offerings of physical movement, stress management, and, if you so choose, a prism through which to reflect on your life.

My journey with yoga began more than 20 years ago in a fitness club in Cambridge, Massachusetts. I am a writer and teacher, and I am fascinated with how to help people change. I was working as the director of the Osteoporosis Awareness Program for the Department of Public Health in Boston. In my work I have noticed that while we all want to be happy and healthy, most of us struggle to make permanent the changes we know will enhance our lives. So, I watch for tools that may help people make shifts. That day in the health club, the curious movements of my first yoga class were physically challenging, but they caught my attention and interest. It was my first taste of what was to become a lifelong personal and professional pursuit.

I have studied with many talented yoga teachers: Patricia Walden who taught me the gift of precision and alignment; then the Kripalu Center for Yoga & Health, with its embrace of compassionate self-acceptance; and later, the master poetess of the internal body, Barbara Benagh, in Boston. Barbara led me deep inside my body, and got me to relax a tiny muscle behind my right kidney that I'd never knew existed—ooh, aah. Bhavani Maki in Kauai coaxed me deep into the devotional practice of vigorous flow yoga. I have settled back at Kripalu, where I have found life mentors, teachers, colleagues, and a home in various forms ever since.

This Eastern practice has informed me physically, mentally, emotionally, personally, and professionally in ways I could not have imagined when I was a 30-year-old registered dietitian nutritionist taking my first yoga class. It has enhanced my life in countless ways.

Since that day in the gym, yoga has ebbed and flowed throughout my life. For periods of time I have wandered away from my mat, but I always make my way back. And that seems to be fine with my yoga practice—it welcomes me back and the exploration begins again. I am not the lithe yogini (female practitioner) I was when I began 20 years ago. I am not immune to the side effects of aging (drat!). But, I know that without this practice, my physical body and certainly my mind would not be the optimistic, strong, creative, and curious place it most usually is. Yoga helps me to ride the waves of my life and relax into what might otherwise be more alarming or upsetting developments.

As my yoga path unfolded, so did my professional career as an integrative registered dietitian nutritionist. For more than 20 years, I have had the honor of working with thousands—maybe hundreds of thousands—of people aiming to improve their health by improving their lifestyles. When Dr. Lisa Nelson came to Kripalu as its director of medical education, I was impressed by her down-to-earth, common sense style of doctoring, and how easily she related to the guests in programs there. We found in our work together a shared mission of reducing the suffering of those who struggle with chronic disease, and we both aim to reduce that suffering by helping people commit to making small doable changes and practicing those changes regularly over time. Over and over I see people make small improvements in their lifestyles, and when those changes are practiced regularly (not perfectly), transformative change in health often follows. The exercises and ideas in this book (with diabetes-specific medical considerations thanks to Dr. Nelson) are designed to help you make those small changes that over time can add up to transformation.

Annie

Also by Annie B. Kay

Every Bite Is Divine (Life Arts Press, 2007)

Yoga and Meditation: Tools for Weight Management
(Wolf Rinke Associates, 2006. Second Edition, 2010)

Introduction

This book is a practical guide developed for people with diabetes and prediabetes. It provides an accessible approach to yoga that can help you manage your diabetes by improving your lifestyle.

In the first chapter we will explore what the science suggests are the benefits of yoga for people with diabetes and prediabetes. We'll explain how yoga makes you feel better and can help you delay or avoid a diagnosis of diabetes. We hope the science makes sense and motivates you to try and practice yoga.

We'll describe just what the practice of yoga is, and what you need to know if you have diabetes to prepare for a safe and effective experience. If you encounter a word or term you don't recognize, we've included a glossary to help with yoga lingo and medical terms. Chapter 3 will describe and illustrate the postures, complete with easy modifications and tips for those with diabetes so that you can make each posture your own safely and effectively. Postures selected include those that practitioners and health professionals agree are helpful for people with diabetes and prediabetes.

If you have medical complications from diabetes, we have included ideas on how to modify a yoga practice safely and effectively for your needs. Remember to speak with your doctor or other member of your medical team about changes to your lifestyle, including beginning a yoga practice. This is particularly important if you have complications that may limit your movement, or for which special precautions are needed. For each posture, you will see the basic alignment, and how to deepen and develop the posture as you become stronger and more flexible.

Chapter 4 will help you assemble postures into a personal program, and provides guidance on how to safely and effectively build your program over time. There is a program for everyone! If you haven't moved much lately, there is a 10–15 minute program for you. When you are ready for more, there is a full 30-minute program. If you have gestational diabetes, there is a program for you. Back pain or fatigue? There are programs for that.

Chapter 5 will discuss how to weave yoga into your life. We hope to motivate you to learn what you need to keep practicing even when you aren't perfect (none of us is, by the way), and how your yoga practice can support the shift to healthy living.

I hope this book launches you on a journey of self-discovery. May you discover the gentle power of your breath and learn how it can change your body and your mind in a positive way. I hope you find the joy of movement that is your birthright. Should the fire of yoga ignite you, I hope that spark grows into a flame that fuels your fullest, deepest life. May your practice bring you happiness, health, and the experience of being your own true self.

Annie

Chapter 1
Yoga for Diabetes

The part can never be well unless the whole is well.

—PLATO

Would you like to learn a program that can help you manage stress, feel better, and facilitate other lifestyle changes that can help you better manage your diabetes?

Our modern lives are overflowing with commitments to family, work, and community. The price of our hectic schedules too often includes health problems. If this scenario sounds familiar, a yoga practice may help. This ancient practice, with roots in Eastern spiritual tradition, is enjoying a groundswell of interest. Recent research revealing just how yoga may benefit health has the attention of the medical establishment. For people with any type of diabetes, the practice of yoga is a tool that can potentially help improve your entire lifestyle.

Diabetes: An Integrative Lifestyle Condition

The development of type 2 diabetes is closely linked to excess body weight and a sedentary lifestyle. While type 2 diabetes can run in families, genes do not entirely predict who will develop the disease. In fact, lifestyle may be a bigger contributor to the development of type 2 diabetes than family history. A 2001 study in the New England Journal of Medicine showed that women who followed a "low-risk lifestyle" (meaning they followed a healthy diet, maintained a body mass index of less than 25, did not smoke, and exercised 30 minutes daily) were 90% less likely to be diagnosed with type 2 diabetes than women who did not fit this lifestyle pattern. This finding held true regardless of family history.

Therein lies the good news: If something in your lifestyle is contributing to your diabetes, then something in your lifestyle can address it.

—DR. LISA NELSON, DIRECTOR OF MEDICAL EDUCATION, KRIPALU CENTER FOR YOGA & HEALTH

This study was confirmed by a longitudinal, multi-year, multi-center interventional study called The Diabetes Prevention Program (DPP). The DPP showed that people at high risk for diabetes (prediabetes) who were able to follow a low-fat, low-calorie diet and exercise 150 minutes per week were able to reduce the risk of progressing to full-blown type 2 diabetes by 58%. For people over the age of 60, this risk reduction was even more striking, at 71%. Later analyses of the DPP even showed that some participants were able to reverse their prediabetes, with blood sugars falling back into the normal range.

When we talk about lifestyle in this book, we are primarily referring to what and how you eat, how you move, handle stress, and cultivate resiliency, as well as the quality of your rest, relaxation, and sleep.

Overweight and obesity refer to excess weight that increases a person's risk of experiencing poor health. According to the U.S. Centers for Disease Control and Prevention (CDC), an adult with a body mass index (BMI) of between 25 and 29.9 is considered overweight (for Asian-Americans, a BMI of 23 or more increases the risk of developing type 2 diabetes). A BMI of 30 or higher is considered obese. While BMI is widely used and relates to body fat, it does not directly measure body fat or other weight-related indicators of health. It is just one indicator. Is there a better measure? Your waist circumference (WC) may be more predictive of weight-related health issues. Together, these two measures may give you an accurate estimate of your weight status.

Here are links from the CDC to help you measure your BMI and WC.

ADULT BMI CALCULATOR:
www.cdc.gov/healthyweight/
assessing/bmi/adult_bmi/english_bmi_
calculator/bmi_calculator.html

ASSESS YOUR WEIGHT:
www.cdc.gov/healthyweight/
assessing/Index.html

Yoga: An Integrative Lifestyle Practice

People practice yoga in different ways for different reasons, including fitness, stress management, and as a spiritual practice. Recently, researchers have discovered more about just how yoga's collection of benefits translates into better health.

While the science of yoga for diabetes is still young, there are now several studies, published in peer-reviewed medical journals, that suggest clear improvements for people with diabetes. Findings from these small but high-quality, randomized, controlled clinical trials have shown significant improvements in blood sugar levels as well as improvements in lipid profiles, blood pressure, body weight, and oxidative stress (a metabolic imbalance) in partici-

pants who practice yoga and meditation on a regular basis.

Science has shown that elements of yoga, namely the mind-body practices of physical movement, yoga breathing, deep relaxation, and meditation, help to manage stress and can be part of a lifestyle that may improve blood sugar levels. While these elements are clearly beneficial, to split the aspects of the full practice in order to study it is a bit of an East-West conundrum. Despite the research challenges, high-quality studies illuminating just how and why yoga is helpful for people with diabetes are taking place at major universities around the world. Research has found that regular yoga practice can improve one's lifestyle, mind, and body; the graphic below illustrates how.

HOW YOGA CAN IMPROVE DIABETES

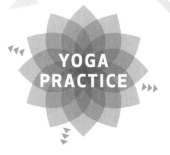

CHANGES IN LIFESTYLE
PHYSICAL ACTIVITY ▲
HEALTHY DIET ▲

YOGA PRACTICE

CHANGES IN YOUR BODY
BODY WEIGHT ▼
BLOOD PRESSURE ▼
CHOLESTEROL ▼
GLUCOSE LEVEL ▼

CHANGES IN YOUR MIND
MOOD ▲
LEVEL OF STRESS ▼
SELF-EFFICACY ▲
QUALITY OF LIFE ▲

Source: Adapted from: *A review of yoga programs for four leading risk factors of chronic diseases.* Yang K. Evidence Based Complementary and Alternative Medicine. 4:487-91. 2007

HOW CAN YOU COPE WITH STRESS?

Having too much stress without managing it can undermine your ability to manage your diabetes. Stress can quickly increase blood sugar levels, undermine your diet, and over time can have a negative impact on your immune, digestive, and other body systems.

The effects of stress tend to build up over time. You can take practical steps to maintain your health and outlook. The following are some tips that may help you to cope with stress:

- **Start and maintain a regular program** to help you cope with stress in your life and the demands of living with diabetes. Your program may incorporate meditation, yoga, tai chi, or other gentle exercises. Prayer and participating in your religious or spiritual practice may also be helpful.

- **See your health-care providers** for your diabetes, any new health problems, and routine checkups.

- **Reach out to and stay in touch with the people in your life** who can provide emotional and other support.

- **Ask for help from friends, family, and community or religious organizations** to reduce stress due to work burdens or family issues, such as caring for a loved one and caring for your diabetes.

- **Practice recognizing signs of your body's response to stress**, such as difficulty sleeping, increased alcohol and other substance use, being easily angered, feeling depressed, and having low energy.

- **Set priorities.** Decide what must get done and what can wait, and learn to say no to new tasks if they are putting you into overload.

- **Note what you have accomplished** at the end of the day, not what you have been unable to do. If things don't go as well as you had hoped in managing your diabetes on a given day, remember that you don't have to be perfect. If you can take some time to think about what got in the way of managing your diabetes, and what you might try next time a similar barrier gets in the way, you are doing just great. Learn from what doesn't work and make a new plan. What can you do to make it easier?

- **Exercise regularly.** Thirty minutes per day of gentle walking can help boost mood and help you better handle stress.

- **Schedule regular times for healthy and relaxing activities.**

- **Seek help from a qualified mental health-care provider** if you are overwhelmed, feel you cannot cope, have suicidal thoughts, or are using drugs or alcohol to cope.

If you or someone close to you is in crisis, call the toll-free, 24-hour National Suicide Prevention Lifeline at 1-800-273-TALK (1-800-273-8255).

Adapted from the National Institute of Mental Health's fact sheet on stress.

Specific Benefits and New Insights

Yoga is itself flexible; it is a tool. As you learn the postures in this book and begin or deepen your practice, you might notice the ways your practice works within and upon your life. Let's take a deeper look at the key reasons why yoga is so helpful for people with diabetes.

Yoga is gentle movement

Let's face it—not everyone with diabetes is ready to don spandex or start running a road race. If you haven't exercised much lately beyond chasing your children or climbing the stairs to your apartment, the gentle stretches of yoga can be a way to invite more movement into your life. The risk of living a sedentary lifestyle is clear: Insufficient movement is associated with nearly every chronic disease.

Modern technology has made physical movement less necessary. Thanks to the Internet and personal computers, you can now work, shop, socialize, and be a fully productive member of society without ever getting off your couch.

Some styles of yoga are more challenging and vigorous than others. If you encounter a class that is too much, don't give up. With the growth of skilled yoga teachers, classes are everywhere, including in your own living room via television or the Internet. Your practice can be modified for your body shape and fitness level, and

PHYSICAL ACTIVITY: THE MAGIC PILL FOR CHRONIC DISEASE

According to the U.S. Centers for Disease Control and Prevention, regular physical activity is one of the most important things you can do for your health. It has been shown to help:

- manage your weight
- keep weight off after you lose it
- reduce your risk for heart disease
- reduce your risk for type 2 diabetes and metabolic syndrome
- reduce your risk for some cancers
- strengthen your bones and muscles
- improve your mental health and mood
- decrease your risk for Alzheimer's disease
- improve your ability to prevent falls
- increase your chances of living longer

you can progress at your own pace. The most important thing is to get started, and to practice at least a little bit—even for 10 minutes—regularly.

Yoga isn't a "sporty" sport: It's come as you are. For most practitioners, it is a quiet time for simple self-reflection. While yoga is generally gentle, athletes also find it helpful. Many athletes complain of tight muscles, and stretches can help warm up and re-lengthen tight overworked muscles. It "gets the kinks out." Yoga breathing is also popular for athletes, offering them better mental focus and the efficiency that comes with the ability to use your breathing for performance.

Yoga makes you feel good

When you do yoga, you breathe more deeply, stretch your muscles, and shift your attitude. Each of these elements of the practice can make you feel better.

To understand how conscious breathing makes you feel good, let's step back and take a look at your whole nervous system. Your nervous system is subdivided into a central and peripheral nervous system. The peripheral nervous system is divided into two parts: the somatic, having to do with sensation and voluntary movement; and the autonomic nervous system, or ANS. The ANS regulates the involuntary processes in your body: those bodily functions you don't need to think about them for them to happen. This includes your digestive organs processing food you eat, the beating of your heart, movement of your lungs, and other involuntary actions. The autonomic nervous system includes the sympathetic (fight or flight) and the parasympathetic (calming and recovery) systems.

While it seems these two sides work in opposition, when in healthy balance they work together to keep you well and reacting appropriately to things around you. In our busy modern lives, however, many people are in a constant state of fight-or-flight activation. Constant sympathetic activation might also be called chronic stress. Yoga helps to release chronic stress and ease your body into recovery mode.

Breathing in a specific way—yoga breathing—supports this recalibration process. Breathing is one of the only physiological functions that is both voluntary and involuntary. You can choose to change the way you breathe, but if you stop paying attention to it, you don't stop breathing. This aspect of breathing is why many yogis (people who practice yoga) consider it a vehicle between your mind and body.

The relationship between breath and emotion is complex and continues to be a hot area of research, though the yogis have been talking about that relationship for thousands of years. We all know what a sharp intake of breath means: that we are surprised or frightened. As it turns out, you can calm your mind by calming your breath. Functional MRIs give a glimpse of how yoga may rebalance brain activity by demonstrating a shift from a fight-or-flight pattern (emotional stress lights up the amygdala of the brain) to a more balanced one (the prefrontal cortex, where complex reasoning occurs).

In yoga, the breath is deeply tied to your energy level and indeed your overall life force. We will dive deeper into yoga breathing practices in Chapter 2.

Why does it feel good to stretch? Endorphins are neuroendocrine (nerve-hormone) factors in your body that, among other things, create the sense of relaxation and well-being that many people experience after practicing yoga. Stretching is one way to trigger the release of endorphins from your pituitary gland (a gland in your brain that secretes hormones that regulate homeostasis). Endorphins plug into receptors on the cells of your central nervous system and make you feel good.

How does yoga help shift your attitude? It's all about the power of pause. Yoga and other wisdom traditions of the East cultivate your observing, less reactive mind, often called your witness. When you learn to activate this viewpoint, it tends to help you respond to life's inevitable problems in a calmer, less emotionally hair-triggered way. Yoga and contemplative practices also include an attitude of nonjudgmental awareness. That is, you practice not labeling things in your world (and even parts of your body) as good or bad. The more you take a break from judging, the more room there seems to be for gratitude and appreciation. In the emerging science of positive psychology, these two emotions are strongly linked to overall happiness.

Yoga balances your lifestyle from the inside out

Your body is a complex collection of systems interwoven into a dynamic whole. If you live an overall happy and healthful life, each of your systems tends to flow toward overall balance.

The movements of yoga make you more aware of the alignment of bones in your skeletal system, from the central axis of your spine to the major joints, down to the small bones in your hands and feet. Good posture and alignment tend to make you feel and operate better. How your skeleton moves in concert with your muscles and your connective tissue (fascia) becomes more apparent. While we are all asymmetric, your practice may point the way to coming into healthier alignment.

Your central nervous system, respiratory system (having to do with breath), endocrine (glands that produce hormones), cardiovascular, and digestive system are all impacted by the movement and positions of the postures. The grounding, expansion and stretch, the slow rhythmic breath, and the mental practice of yoga all tend to make you feel well (which is not to say the journey is free of discomfort). As you become more aware of the systems of your body and how they interact, your brain is also undergoing positive change. Feeling better tends to make positive change easier, and before you know it, you are experimenting with other kinds of healthier changes.

Yoga can help you keep your blood sugar in your target range

Can you begin to see that yoga has a number of potential benefits for people with diabetes? It multitasks! Because it is exercise, yoga improves insulin sensitivity.

When your liver and muscle cells become more sensitive to insulin, this allows glucose (sugar) to enter cells from the bloodstream, which helps you reach your blood sugar targets.

By increasing muscle mass through strengthening poses, yoga can improve your metabolism, helping you maintain a healthy body weight. Studies suggest that regular practice helps normalize blood pressure and cholesterol levels. By inducing a feeling of calm, yoga can lower the release of cortisol, a stress hormone that causes your body to release more glucose. Less unnecessary cortisol means fewer unnecessary elevations in blood sugar.

How much physical activity do you need to help manage your blood sugar? Aim for at least 150 minutes of moderately intense aerobic activity (2 1/2 hours) each week. If you have not been physically active in a while and that much movement feels daunting, start slow (5 or 10 minutes at a time). Over time, work your way up. You may be surprised at the positive spiral of moving more and feeling better, which could allow you to move even more.

Yoga is an excellent form of physical activity that can be adjusted for people at all fitness levels. Now that you have heard about the potential benefits of a yoga practice, are you curious about just what yoga is? Chapter 2 will help get you started.

Chapter 2
The Practice of Yoga

Physical fitness is not only one of the most important keys to a healthy body, it is the basis of dynamic and creative intellectual activity.

—JOHN F. KENNEDY

Ancient Roots

Yoga has a long and rich history. The ancient sage Patanjali codified the philosophy of yoga more than 2,000 years ago in a book called The Yoga Sutras. A collection of deceptively simple yet poetic phrases, the book is a kind of roadmap for the practice of yoga. Patanjali studied people as they logged in years of yoga, and he wrote down what advanced practitioners did and the results of their practices.

In the classic Indian language of Sanskrit, the word *yoga* translates as "union" or "yoking." This is usually thought to mean integrating different aspects of yourself; that is, getting your mind and your physical body walking together on a shared path in the same direction. Patanjali described an eight-limbed path of yoga which includes a particular way of living in balance with the environment and with others, along with practices that cultivate union. The graphic on page 10 outlines the eight-limbed path.

8. SAMADHI
state of yoga

6. DHARANA
focus

7. DHYANA
state of meditation

3. ASANA
pose

4. PRANAYAMA
breath

5. PRATYAHARA
withdrawal of senses

1. YAMAS
restraints

2. NIYAMAS
observances

AHIMSA
non-harming

SAUCHA
cleanliness

SATYA
truth

SANTOSA
contentment

ASTEYA
non-stealing

TAPAS
zeal for yoga

BRAHMACHARYA
self-restraint

SVADHYAYA
self-study

APARIGRAHA
non-hoarding

ISVARA PRANIDHANA
surrender

8 LIMBS OF YOGA

Sanskrit is a complex ancient language that, like Latin, is no longer spoken in daily life. It is the language of yoga, so as yoga becomes more popular it is increasingly common to see Sanskrit words and phrases. In their most correct form, many of the Sanskrit words in this book would contain diacritics (accent or other marks). For simplicity and English readability, we have eliminated them.

It sounds simple enough, but the reality is that in the bustle of modern life, our minds and physical bodies often don't operate in concert. If you have ever multi-tasked—talked on the phone while doing the dishes, or the no-no of texting while driving—you know that combining these activities in order to get more done and save time often results in not doing either task very well. And sometimes things can end quite badly. Just ask the U.S. Department of Transportation, which has found that drivers who text are twice as likely to crash as their less distracted counterparts. One study found that attempting to do more than one thing at a time decreased productivity by as much as 40%. Other studies on multitasking have found that it increases stress.

Focusing on one thing at a time takes practice. People are wonderfully distractible, and our instant-update culture ensures that our attention spans remain short. That's where yoga can come in: Yoga practice can be an antidote to distraction. The combination of activities that are the essential ingredients of yoga have been shown to change bodies and minds in a way that helps people focus, feel better physically and mentally, and even aid in decision-making in other parts of life.

Getting Started

Let using this book and your yoga practice be easy. If it begins to add stress to your life, ease off, and ask yourself how you can make it easier. You can try one posture or one breathing exercise at a time. Or, you can do all the postures and every exercise presented, or something in between. Find a pace that is right for you. Advance your practice slowly and pay attention to how you feel. If you feel fatigued, there is a program in Chapter 4 for that. Helpful props are outlined in Chapter 3.

Find your home yoga space

If you can, find a dedicated space to do your yoga practice. Choose a space where you are most likely to avoid distractions. Make the space as inviting and easy to use as possible. Have music, a box of tissues, water, and anything else you'll need in your space. Make sure the floor or your yoga mat is clear of clutter that could cause falls or injury.

Find a regular time to practice

Choose a regular time to practice, if possible. Even taking 10 minutes each day to practice, perhaps first thing in the morning, can be very beneficial. If you set a time but life gets in the way, no worries, just think of it as an experiment that needs adjustment, and try again. Remember, nobody is perfect, and you don't need to be. The more you experiment with finding those 10 minutes, the more you are likely to benefit. In whatever time you set aside, do what you can, and don't rush to squeeze in more. Make space for yoga in your schedule; mark it on your calendar.

Safety first

The riskiest thing you can do physically is not to move. People who move more feel better. People who move more have fewer aches and pains, not to mention lower rates of diabetes, heart disease, and some cancers. Yoga injuries do exist, but you dramatically decrease your risk of injury by going at your own pace, and resisting the temptation to rush into postures you are not ready for, or deepen into stretches that take you beyond your edge of comfort.

Yoga is a long-term project; there is no hurry. You may get enamored with yoga as you learn to master new poses, but the point of the practice is not so much to be able to fold into interesting shapes or stand on your head. The aim of the practice is to feel good stretching and moving, and to understand yourself and your body better.

Before you begin your practice, talk with your health-care providers. They are likely to encourage you, and they may have suggestions for modifications for your particular medical conditions or diabetes complications. Over time, your health-care provider can track your health, let you know how effective your lifestyle choices and medications are, evaluate any effect your practice may have on your long-term blood sugar management (for instance, adjusting medications), and give you advice on how to make your yoga and other exercise more safe, comfortable, and effective.

Essential Ingredients: Breath, Mind, Body

Yoga has a physical component that features postures aimed at balancing the structure, strength, and flexibility of your body inside and out. Simultaneous to your physical movements, you pay attention to and move with your breath. Breathing is the only bodily function that is both voluntary and involuntary; for example, you can change your breathing pattern by lengthening or deepening each cycle. But if you stop paying attention to it, you don't stop breathing: It continues on its own.

Because of this, in the world of yoga, breathing is considered a vehicle that translates and shuttles messages between the body and the mind. The study of how various ways of breathing impacts your body and emotional state is a hot area of research.

The breathing practice

The Sanskrit word *prana* means "vital energy" or "life force." The practice of *pranayama* involves managing your energy, and it focuses a great deal on your breath. Becoming a student of your own breathing will enable you to use it to calm down in stressful situations, to perk up when you feel low, and to generally feel more energized.

Breath and movements work together. The expansive nature of the inhale can help with the elongating stretch of a muscle or to coax space into a tight joint. Likewise, the releasing nature of the exhale is an opportunity to let go of tension, soften, and relax into deeper comfort even within a challenging posture. The pauses between an inhale and exhale are opportunities to cultivate stillness moment by moment.

Breathing patterns are often established very early in life. Breath training may sound odd: You would think we all know how to do this basic function. In modern life, with its increasing levels of stress, however, learning how to change the pattern of your breath for your health is a practice unto itself. The exercises on the following pages help you explore how your breath, energy level, and emotions interconnect.

The mental practice

An engaged mind is essential for practice. Yoga is not something you can do while multi-tasking or watching television. During your practice, focus your attention inward—on the sensations in your body and on your breath. Your focus is one-pointed. That is, your mind is fully engaged in what is going on in your body. How does each posture and each breath feel? How does it feel beneath your skin? Yoga is a practice of self-exploration, of noticing sensations. Notice where you are asymmetric, for example, and explore why that may be. Be curious. Focus on what is happening right now. We all have a tendency to replay past conversations, for example, or think about the future (such as wondering what to make for dinner). Bring your attention back, over and over and over again, to what is happening right now in your body. No need to punish yourself if you often get distracted. Everyone gets distracted. The more you pull yourself out of the chatter in your mind and quietly observe yourself as though you were a beloved friend, the more "yoga" (or inner union) you will feel. Pay attention to these components, and you are doing yoga even if you are lying still on your mat.

EASY BELLY BREATHING

Easy belly breathing cultivates relaxation and calmness. You can do this kind of breathing exercise either seated or lying down. If you are lying down, either lie comfortably in a bed or on the floor, and let your spine be straight. Or come to a comfortable seated position on a folded blanket or cushion. An erect spine (in a seated position) is preferable as the breath deepens in this practice. Experiment with what works for you. If you lie down for breathing practice, make sure that your breath expands in all directions; let your back and side ribs separate and your back and sides expand along with the front of your body.

1. Begin to notice your breathing. Let your breathing be relaxed and natural. Take five breaths in this way, just noticing. Can you imagine your breath as a soft thread? Follow the thread of your breath in and out of your nostrils, into your lungs, and throughout your body. Do you notice the coolness of the inhale and the warmth of the exhale?

2. Lengthen your spine up through the crown of the head, and begin to deepen your breath without straining or pushing. Invite your breathing to gently deepen. Place one hand on your belly, and one hand on your chest. Begin to breathe into your belly area so that you can see that hand move out with your expanded belly. (You are not literally breathing into your belly. You are inhaling into your lower lungs, which expands the belly out.) Let the hand on your chest stay stationary. As you breathe, feel your hand move forward and back (up and down if you are lying) as the belly fills and empties with breath. Let your exhale get longer without forcing your breath. Smile gently. (2.1, 2.2)

3. After you have practiced this breath for several minutes, release it, and notice how you feel.

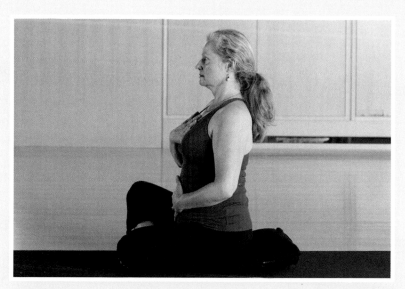

2.1 | Belly Breathing (inhale)

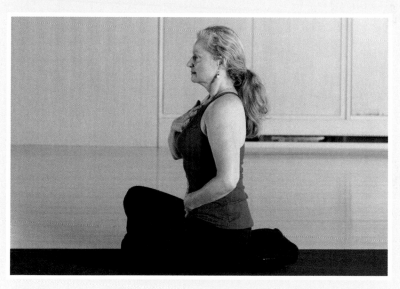

2.2 | Belly Breathing (exhale)

WAVE-SOUNDING BREATH

Wave-sounding breath (called *ujjayi* in Sanskrit) helps to lengthen and deepen your breathing, which facilitates yoga postures that are steady and comfortable. The wave-like sound of this breath also provides a point of focus for the mind.

1. Find a comfortable seated position. Bring one of your hands in front of your face, and exhale onto your palm as if you were fogging a mirror, with a soft "ha-a-a-a." Notice how your throat is slightly pressed back, and keep that position in your throat as you close your lips. (**2.3**)

2. Inhale and exhale, making a soft wave-sounding breath by keeping the glottis (the space around your vocal cords) in your throat slightly pressed toward the back of your throat. So keep your throat in the same position, the fogging-a-mirror position, as you inhale and exhale. Keep your breath smooth and relaxed. If this breathing irritates your throat, you are pushing too hard.

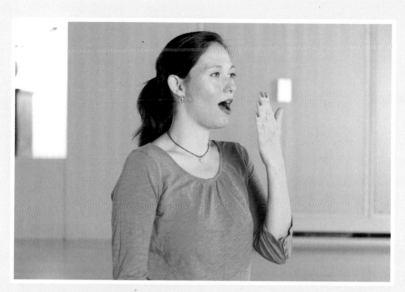

2.3 | Wave-Sounding Breath

ALTERNATE NOSTRIL BREATHING

This sweet breath (called *nadi shodhana* in Sanskrit) is thought to calm and balance the nervous system. It also opens up the nasal passages.

1. Sit in a comfortable upright position (or you can do this breath lying down so long as your spine is straight; consider not having a pillow under your head). Breathe slowly and notice the gentle rhythm of your natural breath.

2. Bend the index and middle finger of your right hand over toward your palm. Keep the other fingers and thumb straight. (**2.4**)

3. Press your right thumb against your right nostril, blocking it off. Place the thumb high enough so that you feel the bone along the side of your nose. Inhale through the left nostril. (**2.5**)

4. Pause, then place the right ring finger over the left nostril, and exhale through the right nostril. Inhale through the right nostril. (**2.6**)

5. Pause, place the thumb back over the right nostril, and exhale through the left.

6. Begin with three cycles of this breath, and increase to 1 to 2 minutes, then work your way up to 10 minutes.

7. Release the hands and breathe easily and smoothly. Notice how your body and your mind feel.

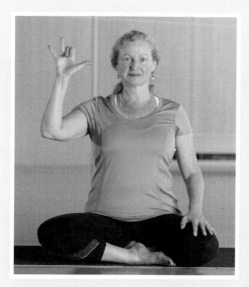

2.4 | Alternate Nostril Breathing

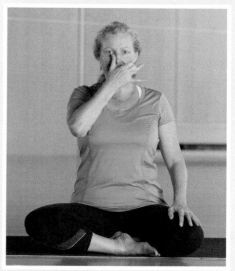

2.5 | Alternate Nostril Breathing

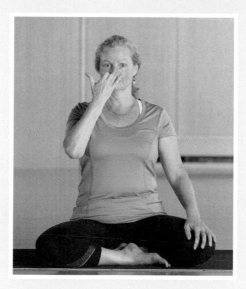

2.6 | Alternate Nostril Breathing

INTENTIONALLY HOLDING YOUR BREATH

Holding your breath (called *kumbhaka* in Sanskrit) is sometimes done at the top of the inhale (internal *kumbhaka*) by retaining your breath or at the bottom of the exhale (external *kumbhaka*) by holding the breath out. Holding your breath for more than a heartbeat or two can be powerful, and this practice is best learned under the guidance of an experienced teacher.

In addition to mental focus, there is a particular attitude in yoga practice. As you practice, aim for nonjudgmental awareness. That is, an attitude of "it's not good, it's not bad, it just is." Mind-chatter, or the noise inside our heads, tends to be negative: We often aren't very kind to ourselves or others. Begin to notice your inner dialogue. By observing just what you are saying to yourself, you can begin to shift that inner critic who prevents you from taking risks or even taking care of yourself, into an inner coach who can encourage you to be the best you can be regardless of what life throws your way.

This is not a "don't worry, be happy" rose-colored-glasses perspective. Rather, it is a technique designed to help ensure that your inner dialogue is true and helpful. A negative inner dialogue reinforces negative feelings. Having negative feelings too much of the time can contribute to not feeling well physically, and can even cause or contribute to depression. Reframing negative self-talk can change the way you feel. How you feel can change the choices you make and the way you behave. Yoga practitioners cite this practice as central to making them feel happy and healthy, and to supporting a mindful, positive, and healthy lifestyle. Use the exercise "Your Internal Dialogue" in Chapter 5 to explore your own self-talk, and begin to reframe it to support making changes that will improve your health.

The physical practice

The physical practice of yoga consists of the postures, or *asanas*. Yoga postures are designed to bring your body into structural alignment. By the time we reach adulthood our bodies reflect decades of physical and emotional living. As a result, one hip may be tighter than the other or one leg a smidgen longer. Everything you do, from driving your car, to your physical activity (or lack of it) and job ends up impacting the shape and function of your body. Working with a yoga teacher who has experience helping people with diabetes or similar physical needs is likely to help guide your progress.

Your bones, which give your body structure, are attached to one another at the joints, and are moved by your muscles. Support your muscles by stretching them wisely and being aware of when you have had enough.

Each yoga practice ends with a period of deep relaxation, in a posture done lying down that is called the corpse pose. This is when your muscles release, your breathing quiets, and your body and your mind relax.

If you are just getting started, remember that yoga is a practice, which means that when you first begin, you might find certain poses or programs difficult. The more you practice the three ingredients of physical movement, breath, and mindfulness, the easier they will be.

How joints work

There are different types of joints in the body. How each joint holds the bones to each other determines the type of movement and stretch the attached muscles do.

The basic types of joints are:

- **Hinge joints:** The knee is a hinge, as are the joints of your fingers, and your elbows—a hinge moves in one plane, straight then bent. You can't make a circle with a hinge joint. Keeping a 90-degree angle provides better support and prevents strain. For example when you bend your knee in a posture, we will remind you to have your knee parallel with (pointing straight over) your three middle toes.

- **Ball-and-socket joints:** Your shoulders and hips have a ball-and-socket configuration, which allows movement in all directions. When you circle your arms up overhead, it's the ball-and-socket of the shoulder that allows that free range of movement. Likewise when you are lying on the floor, you can circle your leg in any direction, thanks to the ball-and-socket of the hip. The mobility of these joints can undermine their stability if used incorrectly.

- **Other types of joints:** Some joints glide bones one over the other, which tends to keep your movement of that joint limited. The tiny joints between your rib bones and spine, for example—they move to accommodate your breathing and digestion, and otherwise keep that central structure stable. There are also joints where a curved bone fits into another curve. Your wrist and the joint that attaches your head to your spine are examples of this type of joint.

Special Considerations for People with Diabetes

If you have complications from diabetes, you can adjust your practice. In this section we describe common complications with ideas on how to accommodate them. See Chapter 3 for specific modifications to your yoga practice and Chapter 4 for recommended programs. If you have uncontrolled hypertension, severe autonomic neuropathy, a history of foot lesions, or unstable proliferative retinopathy, talk to your doctor. You may need a more thorough evaluation before starting a new exercise program.

Are you at risk for hypoglycemia (low blood sugar)?

Low blood sugar is normally defined as less than 70 mg/dL. It may be asymptomatic, or accompanied by the following symptoms:

- Rapid heartbeat
- Weakness and fatigue
- Hunger or nausea
- Feeling shaky, unsteady, or dizzy

MODIFY YOUR YOGA PRACTICE TO ACCOMMODATE DIABETIC COMPLICATIONS AND RELATED HEALTH ISSUES

DIABETES COMPLICATION	AVOID	TRY
Heart disease	• Vigorous practice	• Beginning with gentle practice and work up to moderate level
High blood pressure *Note: defined as greater than 140/90*	• Vigorous practice	• Gentle to moderate practice
Autonomic dysfunction or low blood pressure	• Vigorous practice • Moving quickly between postures	• Gentle to moderate practice • Slow and careful transitions between postures, especially moving between seated or on your back to standing
Peripheral neuropathy	• Practicing barefoot • Prolonged standing postures if your sensation is impaired or if you experience pain	• Practicing with soft shoes or sneakers and socks to protect your feet • Seated or supine (on your back) poses
Peripheral vascular disease	• Prolonged standing postures or vigorous movement	• Gentle to moderate programs that focus on seated and supine postures. Consider using a chair to modify standing postures (see Chapter 3 for more modifications) • Moving carefully between postures
Retinopathy	• Postures where your head is below your heart (forward bends, downward dog) • Vigorous practice	• Standing, seated, or supine postures that keep your head above or even with your heart • Gentle to moderate practice
Low blood sugar *Note: defined as less than 70 mg/dL*	• Exercising if your blood sugar is less than 100 mg/dL, if you take medication that affects insulin levels	• Drink 4 oz of fruit juice • Check your blood sugar after 15–20 minutes • If it is >100 mg/dL it is safe to begin your yoga practice
Arthritis	• Holding postures that flex tender joints, such as downward dog (wrists), warrior poses (knees), or one-legged balance (ankle)	• Warming up with gentle joint rotations prior to practice • Using blocks or other supports to reduce strain on the affected joint (see Chapter 3 for specific modifications)

People who are managing their diabetes without medication ("diet-controlled diabetes") are rarely at risk for this complication. However, people with type 1 diabetes or those with type 2 or gestational diabetes who require insulin (or insulin secretagogues) may experience low blood sugar. If this happens, drink 4 oz of fruit juice or another form of fast-acting carbohydrate (2 tablespoons of raisins or 8 oz of low-fat milk). Wait until your blood sugar is >100 mg/dL and you are feeling well, before starting your yoga practice.

Diabetes medications

Diabetes medications that may cause hypoglycemia (low blood sugar):

All forms of insulin, including Lantus and Levemir, NPH and regular insulin, and rapid-acting agents such as Humalog, Novolog, and Apidra

Oral medications that promote the release of insulin:

Sulfonylureas, such as glipizide (Glucotrol), glyburide (Diabeta), and glimepiride (Amaryl); repaglinide (Prandin) and nateglinide (Starlix); or any combination pills that contain these medications

Medications less likely to cause hypoglycemia:

Metformin (Glucophage), exenatide (Byetta), liraglutide (Victoza), sitagliptin (Januvia), saxagliptin (Onglyza), linagliptin (Tradjenta), and pioglitazone (Actos).

Your safe yoga practice checklist

☐ Check with your health-care provider before starting any new exercise program.

☐ Remember to check your blood sugar before and after exercise and eat a healthy snack if your level is below 100 mg/dL.

☐ Stay hydrated by drinking plenty of water before and after exercising.

☐ Start with a slow or gentle practice.

☐ Slowly increase the amount of time you practice, week by week.

☐ Increase the speed or vigor of your practice as tolerated. Pay attention to how you feel afterwards: are you fatigued, or energized? If you feel pain, excess fatigue or strain, slow down.

☐ A good goal to work toward is 150 minutes of moderate exercise per week.

Check with your health-care team at regular intervals, especially if you notice changes in blood sugar levels or if you gain or lose weight. You may need to adjust your medications to keep your blood sugar, blood pressure, and cholesterol levels in target range.

Chapter 3
Yoga Postures

*Yoga teaches us to cure what need not be endured
and endure what cannot be cured.*

—B.K.S. IYENGAR

The great yogi B.K.S. Iyengar said that when a posture is correct, one feels lightness, freedom. He said that freedom comes when every part of the body is active. "Let us be free in whatever pose we are doing," he said. "Let us be full in whatever we do."

Let each posture in your yoga practice feel easeful, stable, and comfortable. Never press into pain or physical discomfort. If adjusting a posture does not make it comfortable, either continue adjusting or release it. A skilled yoga teacher can also help you develop a stable and comfortable practice.

Begin by reading through the postures described in this chapter, and gently try them out (walls, chairs, and sturdy tables can be wonderful supportive props). Once you feel comfortable with a few postures, you might begin putting them together into a series of postures, or programs. There are a variety of programs included in this book, including flows for beginners and those for more advanced practitioners. We describe particular issues that people with diabetes may experience.

The programs are designed to guide individuals with diabetes to slowly build a safe and effective practice. You can find practice programs outlined in Chapter 4.

Yoga is about being comfortable. Wear loose clothing that you can easily move in, and soft shoes or sneakers if they improve your stability. If you enjoy shopping, you probably already know that yoga outfits are widely available, attractive, and often can be worn throughout the day.

Props

Props support a comfortable alignment and are used as tools to help you deepen your practice. When you use the wall to help balance in your first tree pose, for example, you can then focus on the essence of the posture—the rooting down and upward growth. The posture will then naturally unfold in a safe and supported way. Practicing without props does not necessarily produce a more advanced practice; it's just different. The postures included in this book are ones that yoga and medical experts agree are beneficial to those working with diabetes.

Here are some commonly used yoga props, although none of them is mandatory.

Sticky mat or rug

Yoga mats, made from rubber and other materials, help prevent your feet from slipping on the floor, especially in standing

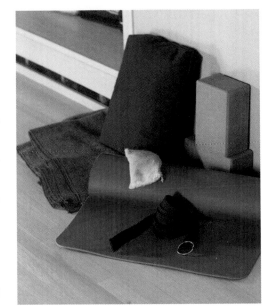

3.1 | Props

postures. Mats and rugs also protect and cushion knees and other joints that may otherwise bump or scrape on the floor. Yoga is usually done barefoot. But, if you have difficulty balancing with bare feet, wear sneakers or soft shoes with good support to enhance your stability.

Cushion or blanket

Having something to sit on will make your practice more comfortable and effective. A folded wool or cotton blanket can be adjusted to the height you need for a particular posture. Experiment with cushions and other soft items. You may enjoy a light blanket over you for supine (lying down) postures, and for relaxation.

Blocks and wedges

A sturdy yoga block is a useful tool that you can sit on or use in standing postures where your hands reach toward the floor. Blocks are made of wood, cork, or other materials. There is an assortment of shapes and sizes of foam props, including wedges, which can be particularly helpful for people with wrist issues. You can also experiment with using household items (that epic novel may make a handy prop when you are not reading it). Make sure all your props are sturdy enough to hold your weight and stable enough to support you as you move.

Straps

Yoga straps can be helpful when your arms need to be just a little longer to reach your toe or foot. With a strap, the back can stay in safe and proper alignment and you can still get the stretch you are after. Straps are also used to help hold your body as you relax into a hip opening or other postures.

Tables, chairs, the wall, and other household items

If you need a prop, get creative and look around. Books, tables, couches, and other things already in your home may be the perfect props. Make sure your makeshift prop is up to the task before using it to bear your full weight.

Postures

Postures in this book include:

- Table
- Cat and dog
- Child
- Mountain
- Half moon
- Standing forward fold
- Triangle
- Tree
- Warrior 1
- Warrior 2
- Warrior 3
- Extended side angle
- Downward facing dog
- Cobra
- Seated forward fold
- Seated spinal twist
- Cobbler
- Hero
- Bridge
- Abdominals
- Wind-relieving
- Legs up the wall
- Corpse

TABLE
(hands and knees)

Table is a stable foundational posture for exploring movement along the spine and central body. If you have wrist pain, modify the posture by forming a fist, and/or use a blanket under your hands for cushion. (**3.3**) If the knees are uncomfortable, use a blanket under them.

1. Come onto hands and knees.

2. Place your hands directly beneath the shoulders, fingers wide, middle finger pointing forward. Press into the hands at the base of the fingers, and even out the weight throughout the palm. Feel the connection of your hands to the floor. (**3.2**)

3. Bring your knees directly below your hips.

4. Lightly engage your belly, drawing it toward the spine. Feel your tailbone drop (imagine having a tail like a dog or cat, and let your tail drop between your legs).

5. Roll your shoulders down your back and away from the ears, so your shoulder blades move toward one another, which allows your chest to open.

6. Lengthen through the crown of the head.

7. Press through your hands and breathe deeply, feeling the wave of breath and how it undulates the central body. Gently lengthen the spine and engage the belly by drawing the belly button toward the spine. Engaging or activating your belly muscles helps to keep your spine straight as you lengthen.

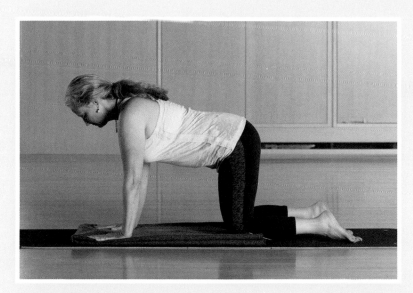

3.2 | Table

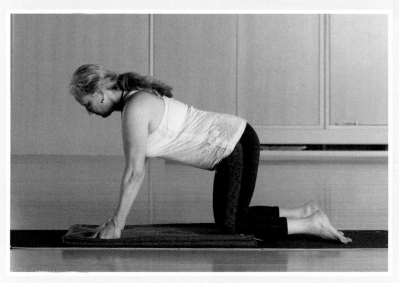

3.3 | Table

CAT AND DOG
(hands and knees, moving spine)

Cat and dog breathing creates a wave of gentle movement around the spine.

1. Come into table position.

2. On an inhale, let your chest widen and draw forward as your belly drops a bit and your tailbone rolls up toward the sky in a dog position. Wag your tail, and then come to stillness. (**3.4**)

3. On an exhale, press the belly up toward the sky, letting the head drop down toward the floor and the tailbone roll under like a Halloween cat. (**3.5**)

4. Continue this breath slowly for 10–15 rounds. Can you feel areas along your spine where there is less movement? Are there areas that feel a little stuck? As you move, let your breath create space along the spine. All you have to do is become aware of the parts of your spine that are not participating, and that tends to begin the process of calling those parts back into movement. Feel a fluid wave of movement. Explore the ways the spine can undulate in this supported breath-filled stretch.

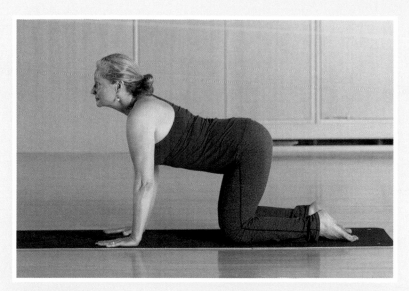

3.4 | Cat and Dog

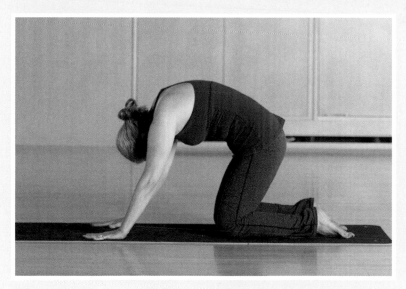

3.5 | Cat and Dog

CHILD
(hips to feet forward release)

Child allows you to be held by the earth. Your breathing gently stretches your back body.

1. Begin in table posture.

2. Inhale, and on the exhale, relax your hips back toward your heels. (**3.6**)

3. Find a comfortable position for your arms. Rest your head in your hands, or extend arms overhead along the floor, or tuck arms back, hands resting on or near your feet.

4. If you do not come down fully into this forward fold, use props such as cushions or blankets to find a comfortable position. (**3.7**)

VARIATIONS: WARM-UP POSES

Nearly any posture, if done with ease and a gentle exploration of your full range of motion, can be a good warm-up. As you stand, slowly and gently circling the shoulder joints and wrists, circling the hips, bending into the elbows, and moving each joint in the hands and fingers to their full range will warm up the upper-body joints. If you are lying on the floor, you can explore the range of motion of the lower-body joints by lifting the feet toward the ceiling and circling each ankle, then flex and point the foot, bending into each knee, then circle your legs to explore the hip joints.

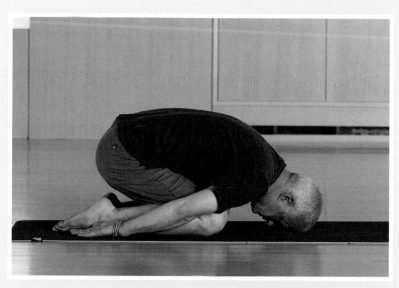

3.6 | Child

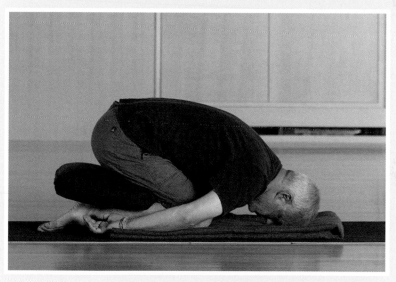

3.7 | Child (with props)

MOUNTAIN
(even standing)

Mountain pose brings you into balanced evenness and makes you more aware of your body's natural alignment as well as proper yoga alignment. This foundational yoga alignment is of benefit in all other postures.

1. Create a solid base for your posture with proper foot alignment. Stand with your feet directly under your hips, toes facing forward, and your second and third toes in line with the knees and hips. Notice if your feet tend to point outward or inward in your natural stance, and point your feet forward.

2. If you can, lift and spread the toes, so that you can see a bit of floor between each toe. This may take practice. Can you press down through the ball and heel of the foot, inner and outer corners? Lift your arches as the foot presses down. Rock forward and back to get the feel of being balanced evenly, both rooting down and lifting up through the legs.

3. Engage the muscles of your legs. Get the feeling of hugging your muscles to the bone. Lift evenly, front, back, and each side of the leg. Lift your kneecaps, aiming for stability without hardness in the joint.

4. Imagine the pelvis lifting off the legs. Drop the tailbone down, belly gently engaged, and create space between the pelvis and ribcage.

5. Lengthen your spine. Collarbones widen away from one another as the shoulders draw down the back without collapsing the back ribs. Create space inside your pelvis, belly, and chest with your breath, intention, and small movements of the muscles and bones. (**3.8**)

6. Stretch the arms downward, and then let them be relaxed at your sides.

7. Lengthen the neck without straining. Let the head be light and float at the top of the spine. Relax your face and soften your eyes.

8. Stay here for 10–15 easy breaths.

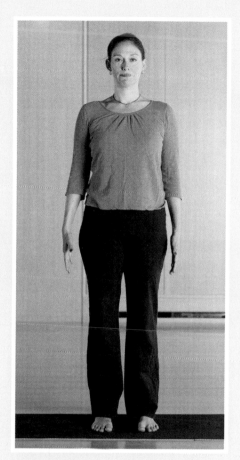

3.8 | Mountain

AWARENESS:

Notice your natural alignment. No one is perfectly symmetrical (identical on the right and left side, for example), and as we go through life, our bodies tend to become more asymmetric. One alignment issue impacts another. For example, if your right foot rolls outward, it is likely that your right knee rolls to the right and the right hip may either compensate or roll to the side. Initially, don't worry about fixing your alignment. First, notice it. As you relax and find comfort in the yoga posture, get curious about your body. Focus on the sensations you feel in your body, adjusting to bring more life and freedom into the posture. Explore the dance of being relaxed and alert and engaged all at the same time. You are centered, even, balanced: Let your nose be directly over your belly button. Shoulders are in alignment with hips, and with knees and feet. Can you lift evenly though your body? Find the sense of balancing one body part atop another. Root down to lengthen up.

HALF MOON
(lateral standing stretch)

Standing lateral stretch awakens the torso and cultivates space in and around the ribs and central organs and tissues.

1. Begin in mountain, with your feet hip-width apart.

2. Exhale, and on the inhale, extend the arms out to the side then up overhead. Relax the shoulders down the back. If you can, bring the palms together overhead. (**3.9**) Feel free to bend either elbow if that is more comfortable. Arm variations include holding one elbow with the opposite hand. Remember the primary stretch is in the side torso, so let the arm position simply be comfortable. (**3.11, 3.12**)

3. Exhale, and on the inhale, lengthen out of the waist. On an exhale, press the hips to the left as your trunk (or torso) lengthens up and dives to the right. Keep the shoulders rolling down the back, both feet evenly pressing into the floor, legs are active. Breathe and stretch into the side body. Hold for two to three breaths, working up to five to eight breaths per side. (**3.10**)

4. Exhale, and on the inhale come back to standing. Exhale the arms down.

5. Repeat on the second side.

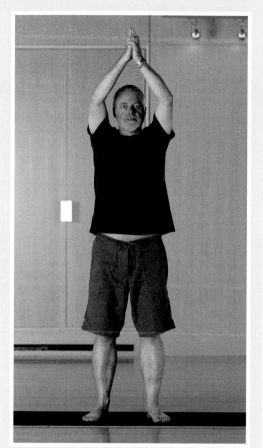

3.9 | Half Moon

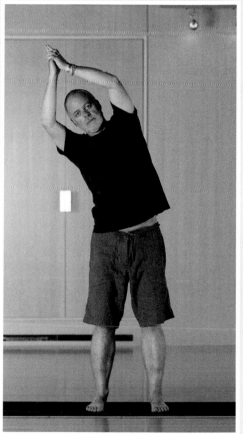

3.10 | Half Moon

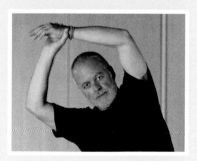

3.11 | Half Moon (arm variations)

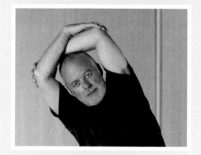

3.12 | Half Moon (arm variations)

STANDING FORWARD FOLD

This stretch can be done passively for relaxation, or actively for a deep stretch throughout the back body. Diabetic retinopathy, high blood pressure, and glaucoma may be aggravated in a posture where your head is closer to the floor than your heart. If you have one of these conditions, either skip this posture (both versions), or modify it by resting your hands on a wall, and bending the hips only to 90 degrees, so that your head is at the same height as your torso or above. This is similar to variation 1 of downward facing dog (page 57). Pregnant women should practice forward folds and inversions only under the guidance of a skilled teacher. Safety first. If in doubt, try another posture.

VERSION 1: PASSIVE STRETCH

1. Stand with feet hip-width apart. Soften the knees and look down to make sure that the feet are pointing forward, knees over heels. Reach the arms overhead, clasping opposite elbows. Roll the shoulders down the back.

2. Inhale and lengthen up at the same time you root (press) down. On the exhale, soften (slightly bend) the knees, and take the trunk and arms forward and down, bending at the hip. (**3.13**)

3. Relax the neck and head down. Keep the torso lengthening evenly and the weight even on each foot. Release your hands to your shins or the floor if that is more comfortable. Begin with taking 10 long smooth breaths, relaxing more deeply with each exhale. Breathe into your low back. Over time, increase to 2–3 minutes.

4. To release, engage the belly, slightly bend the knees, press through the feet, and lengthen through the crown of your head as you come back to standing. (**3.14**)

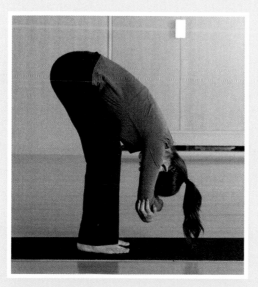

3.13 | Standing Forward Fold (passive)

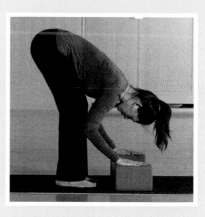

3.15 | Standing Forward Fold (passive)

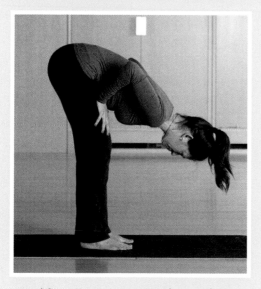

3.14 | Standing Forward Fold (passive)

AWARENESS:
Protect your lower back by bending a little at the knees, especially if your back is tight. This is a great way to begin forward folds.

VERSION 2: ACTIVE STRETCH

1. Stand in mountain pose with attention to alignment. Exhale, and on the inhale, reach your arms (stretching through each finger) up overhead, shoulder width apart. Root down through the feet as you engage the belly slightly and lengthen upward.

2. Inhale, and on the next exhale, slowly and gracefully lengthen through the crown of the head as you fold forward, softly bending the knees. Let the hands rest on the floor, or your legs. On an inhale, come to a flat back, rolling the shoulders down the back and keeping the heart/chest open. (**3.16**)

3. On an exhale, fold forward and gently stretch the torso downward. Keep your weight even on the feet. Breathe and notice sensations in the body. Begin with two to three breaths and work up to 10–15 breaths in this posture. To release, root (press) down through the feet, slightly bend the knees, engage the belly, and rise back to standing.

WORKING DEEPER

Once you have more flexibility in the back, slowly straighten the knees, keeping your belly relaxed and moving toward the chest, your lower belly moving toward the thighs.

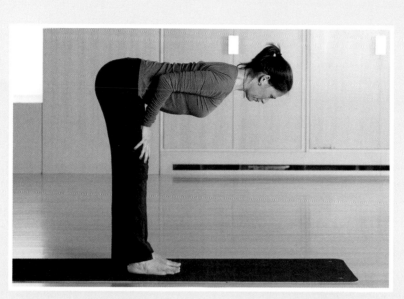

3.16 | Standing Forward Fold (active)

TRIANGLE
(standing side stretch)

This complex posture explores asymmetric stretch alignment anchored with core (trunk or torso) stability and grounding. Do not do this posture if you have had recent surgery or inflammation of your back, legs, or feet. Use caution if you are pregnant (avoid vigorous movement of the abdomen) or have general weakness.

1. Stand in mountain posture. Step the feet approximately 3 feet apart. (If you reach your arms wide, your feet can be the distance of your wrists, or for a gentler posture, closer.) Activate the belly (draw the belly in toward the spine), and drop the tailbone to help lengthen the spine. Exhale, and on the inhale, reach your arms to the side, lifting to shoulder height. You are now in a starfish or five-pointed star position. (**3.17**)

2. Rotate your right foot to 90 degrees. Notice if you can bend you right knee directly over the right foot, and if that does not happen easily, adjust the back foot (you might try stepping forward a bit from the plane of the posture). Then straighten the forward leg. Notice, after your adjustment, if the posture feels more stable. If it does not, keep exploring until it does. Shift the left (back) heel further back than the toes.

3. Root down through the feet, lift the toes to activate the leg, and keep the leg muscles lifting as you relax the toes back to the floor. Re-engage the belly, lengthen the spine, exhale, and on the inhale, reach to the right as if you are reaching across a table. Shift your left hip back. Look down, and notice if your face is in line with your forward foot. (**3.18**)

4. Rotate the trunk so that the right arm is extending toward the sky, and the left arm is reaching down toward earth. (**3.19**) Keep the belly engaged and the legs active for stability.

5. Exhale, and on the inhale, engage the belly, press through the feet, and inhale back to standing. Begin with 10 breaths, and work up to holding this posture for 2–3 minutes on each side.

6. Repeat, reaching to the left.

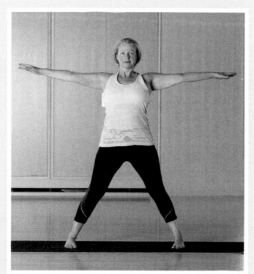

3.17 | Triangle

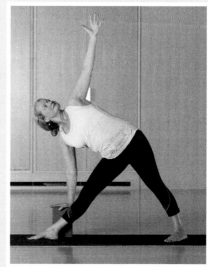

3.19 | Triangle

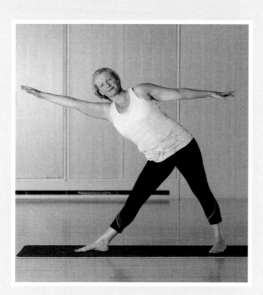

3.18 | Triangle

AWARENESS:

Modify each posture to create stability and comfort. In standing wide-legged postures, the farther the feet are apart, the more vigorous the posture. You might also explore changing the rotation of your feet or direction of your hips to bring more ease. Imagine your triangle posture beginning deep in your engaged abdomen, and your whole body unfurls in a spiral like the petals of a rose. The chest rolls toward the ceiling as the crown of the head reaches forward and the spine lengthens. Your arms and legs rotate externally (while staying stable and pressing into the feet).

TREE
(one-leg balance)

In this posture you learn balance—to stay rooted and strong yet able to sway in the wind like our wise friends the trees. Balance postures are practical training to help prevent falls. Use props like a chair or wall for support as needed. (**3.21**)

1. Stand in mountain pose. Firm the muscles of the left leg and press down through the left foot. Let the right foot become light.

2. Draw the right foot up the left leg, resting it either:
   - at the ankle with toes on the floor for support, or
   - on the calf, or
   - above the knee, or
   - heel to groin.

3. Press the right knee back gently to open the right hip. (**3.20**)

4. Exhale, and on the inhale, extend your arms to the side and then up overhead. Either press the palms together, clasp opposite elbows, or reach in a way that gives the shoulders space.

5. Breathe and extend upward through the torso. Begin by holding the posture while you take 10 breaths, and work your way up to holding the posture for 2–3 minutes. Inhale, and on an exhale release to standing.

6. Repeat on the second side.

WORKING DEEPER
Once your balance is steady, if you would like to challenge yourself, close your eyes in tree posture for a few breaths.

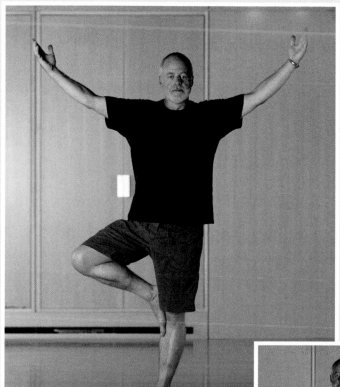

3.20 | Tree

AWARENESS:
In balance postures (as in life balance) there are universal principles. For steady balance:
- Calm your breath;
- Root (press) steadily into the ground;
- Focus your gaze steadily on a point that will not move.

3.21 | Tree (with support)

WARRIOR 1
(standing reach 1)

Warrior strengthens the legs and core, and creates space in the upper body. In this posture, grow your roots to strongly support spreading your wings!

1. Stand in mountain posture at the front of your mat or with space behind you to step back.

2. Step the right foot straight back in line with the right hip. Keep the step narrow enough that the whole back foot can be on the floor. Make sure that the front foot is pointing straight forward. Press down through the feet to feel stable. If you feel unstable, narrow your stance with a smaller step back, and let your feet be a little wider apart from one another.

3. Imagine dropping your tailbone down between your legs as you draw the right hip gently forward, and relax the left hip back, which will square your hips forward. Engage the belly. Feel the bones of the legs rooting down into the earth as the muscles of the legs lift up lightly. (**3.22**)

4. Inhale, and on an exhale, bend into the forward knee until it floats right over the arch of the forward foot. Don't let your knee go beyond the point where this forward shin is perpendicular to the floor.

5. Exhale, and on the inhale, lift and expand your chest as though you could fill it with breath, as you reach your arms upward, keeping the shoulders relaxed down. Keep the lower body grounded and strong as you create space in the spine, shoulder joint and in your attitude. Smile. (**3.23**)

(continued on pg. 48)

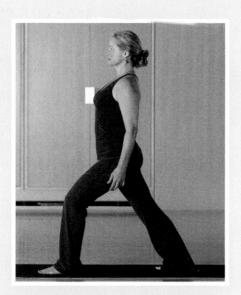

3.22 | Warrior 1

AWARENESS:
Each posture is a dance of intentional effort and surrender to what is. There is rigor and softness. Begin by entering a posture with the most excellent alignment you are able, then notice where you can soften and relax—your jaw, face, toes, inner groin?

3.23 | Warrior 1

6. How can you create more ease in the posture? Is there anything you can let go of and relax—your jaw, your fingers, your eyebrows, toes? Imagine more flow, less push. Begin with holding this posture for five to 10 breaths, and work your way up to 2–3 minutes. Inhale, and on an exhale, release your arms down and step your feet together.

7. Do the posture on the other side, stepping back with the left foot. Between sides, you can place your hands down on the floor and lunge, then step the other foot forward. (**3.24**)

WORKING DEEPER

Work your lunge for strength and balance. The essence of this posture is its lunge—one foot forward with bent knee, one leg reaching back. Lunges have been adopted by the fitness community, and they can be excellent strengtheners for the lower body. Work on strengthening your legs by deepening the lunge; dropping your hips closer to the floor, keeping the forward knee in alignment over the heel, and your back straight. Can the inner groin of your back leg be light and lift toward the ceiling as you extend down through the back heel? Alternatively, work on balance and give the hips more space by lifting the back heel up toward the ceiling.

VARIATION: WARRIOR 3 (BALANCING WARRIOR)

This posture continues to strengthen the legs and core as you develop balance.

1. Begin in Warrior 1. Bow your torso over the forward leg as you strengthen into that leg.

2. Engage your belly and lighten the weight on the back foot.

3. Lift onto the forward leg, extending the back leg straight and in line with the chest and head. Begin by just lifting the back leg up a foot of so off the floor. Place your hands against a wall or on a chair to support you as you build strength. Eventually, the leg and your torso will be parallel with the floor. (**3.25**)

4. When the leg is perpendicular to the floor, even the hips by dropping the hip of the extended leg to be even with the hip of your standing leg.

5. Begin with three to five breaths on each side, and work your way up to 1 minute. To release, lengthen through the crown of your head and reach through your fingers, belly engaged, as you come back to stand and place both feet on the floor.

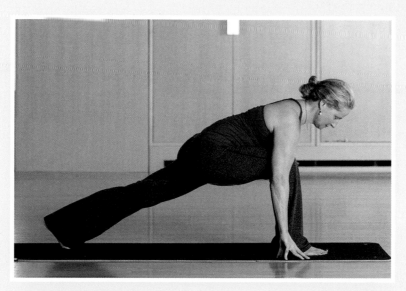

3.24 | Warrior 1 (lunge)

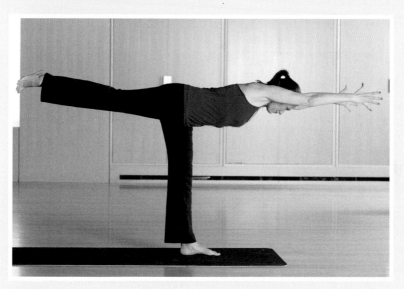

3.25 | Warrior 3

WARRIOR 2
(standing reach 2)

Warrior 2 teaches you how to use your whole being skillfully to make something physically vigorous into something less so. That happens when correct alignment makes this posture more a gentle balance than a muscular holding.

1. Stand at the center of your space, facing sideways.

2. Step the feet about legs width apart. Let the heels be a little (an inch or so) farther apart than the toes. For a gentler posture, narrow your stance. Press through the feet as you draw the muscles of the legs upward and inward toward the bone. Drop the tailbone down as you engage the belly.

3. Rotate the right foot 90 degrees. Spread the toes. If you feel a pull in your left hip and are not able to comfortably bend into the forward knee and keep it aligned over the toes, then step the back foot forward a bit. Square the hips a little (so you face a bit more forward), allowing for more space in the hips and knees. (**3.26**)

4. Bend into the forward knee until the shin is perpendicular to the floor.

5. Exhale, and on the inhale, lift the arms up, reaching forward and back. Relax the shoulders down the back. Inhale, and on the exhale turn to look over the forward fingers. (**3.27**)

6. Now is when you explore the posture to make it more easeful: Can it be more about balance than about muscular strength? Hold the posture for five to 10 breaths and work your way up to 1–2 minutes.

7. Inhale, and on the exhale, release the arms down. Exhale, and on the inhale, straighten into the forward leg and then step the legs back together.

8. Repeat on the left.

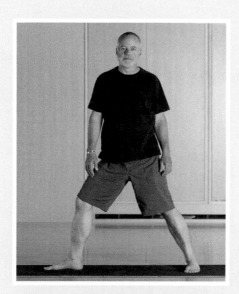

3.26 | Warrior 2

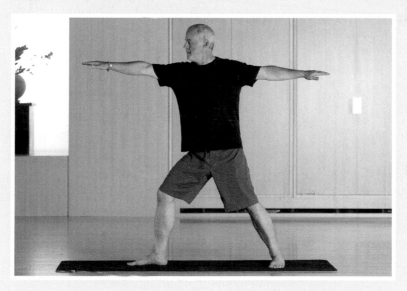

3.27 | Warrior 2

EXTENDED SIDE ANGLE
(standing side stretch 2)

This is a deep side lunge with a twist. Practice this posture to gain strength and flexibility.

1. Stand at the center of your mat in mountain posture, facing sideways.

2. Step the feet hip-width apart, toes a little closer to each other than the heels.

3. Rotate the right foot 90 degrees, so that it faces forward. Press through both feet.

4. Inhale, and on the exhale, bend the forward knee so that it tracks over the forward ankle. Let your shin be perpendicular to the floor. Lightly engage your belly and legs. (**3.28**)

5. Exhale, and on the inhale, reach forward through the right arm to draw your torso to the right.

6. Spread the arms so that you are reaching down with the right and up with the left. Rest your right hand on a block, or on the floor beside your right foot. (**3.29**)

7. Draw your left arm out in front of you and roll you shoulder down the back. This integrates and stabilizes your shoulder. Then, keeping your shoulder integrated, inhale the left arm up alongside your left ear. (**3.30**)

8. Feel the stretch in the line between your left heel and the left hand reaching. Stay active in the belly and allow the top hip to feel light and lifted. Keep the muscles in your legs active as you let the base of the thigh in the bent leg be heavy. Open the chest toward the ceiling. Either look straight ahead, or if it is comfortable, look up. Breathe and relax for five to 10 breaths, working your way up to 1–2 minutes per side.

9. Exhale, and on the inhale, engage the belly to lift you to standing as you straighten into the forward leg.

10. Repeat on the second side.

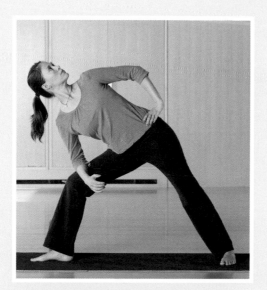

3.28 | Extended Side Angle

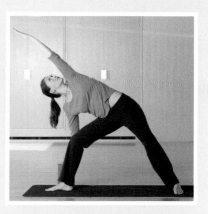

3.30 | Extended Side Angle

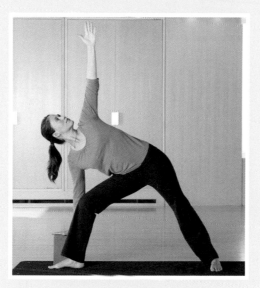

3.29 | Extended Side Angle

AWARENESS:

In a stronger pose like this one, keep your breath light and steady, work at your own pace, and be your own watchdog for strain. If your breath becomes uneven, soften the posture or release it. Work a deeper posture like you are getting to know a powerful, interesting new friend.

DOWNWARD FACING DOG
(lifted table)

An arm balance and partial inversion, down dog is an elongating active stretch of the torso and legs that also serves as a restful pause within an active practice. Do not do this posture if you have had recent injury of the hands, wrists, or shoulders, or if you have diabetic retinopathy, glaucoma, or uncontrolled high blood pressure. If you have one of these conditions, you may try variation 1; be sure to keep your head in line with or above your torso. This will prevent you from increasing pressure to your head or eyes. For people with larger bodies, particularly if your arm strength is low, try the modifications presented first.

1. Begin in neutral table position, hands under shoulders and knees under hips. Spread your fingers wide, with middle fingers parallel. Root through the index finger and thumb, and press gently through the knuckles. Let your wrists be light.

2. Let the upper arm rotate outward so that the shoulders are wide and the chest open.

3. Look forward and gently smile. Inhale, and on the exhale, press into the hands and lift the hips up toward the ceiling. Keep the knees bent at first so that you can emphasize lengthening your spine. Press the floor away with your hands to give the arms a stretch. Keep your shoulders stable by rolling them down the back and away from the ears. (**3.31**)

4. Bend into one knee and press the opposite heel to the floor to open the back of the legs. Repeat, alternating heels. Then, release both heels evenly toward the floor.

5. If it's comfortable, align your ears with your arms, gently lengthening the neck. If it is more comfortable to drop the head and just let the neck relax, you can do that.

6. Press the hips toward the back of the room. Draw the belly button toward the spine.

7. Keep the weight even on both hands and feet. Keep sending your upper leg bones back to lengthen the spine.

8. Breathe in the posture for 10–12 breaths, working up to 2–3 minutes.

9. Inhale, and on the exhale, release the knees back to the floor.

(continued on pg. 56)

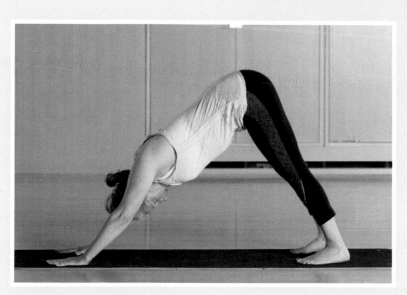

3.31 | Downward Facing Dog

If you are unable to support your weight on your arms, modify the pose in one of the following ways. These modifications can build strength in the arms and upper body gently and safely.

VARIATION 1: DOWNWARD DOG AGAINST THE WALL

1. Face a wall, standing about one-half leg's distance from the wall. Press into your feet, and activate your belly by drawing it in toward the spine.

2. Reach your hands forward and place them shoulder-width apart, on the wall. Press into your hands, and let your shoulders integrate into your back by rolling them back and down.

3. Begin to drop your head between your arms as you lengthen your back through your tailbone.

Engage your belly, and take a step back—a leg's distance from the wall—if your belly and arm strength can hold you. Press into your hands, reach your hips back, and breathe for 10 breaths, slowly working your way into a minute or two. (**3.32**)

4. Engage the belly, exhale, and on the inhale, step forward, coming back to a standing position.

VARIATION 2: DOWNWARD DOG ON A CHAIR

1. Place a sturdy chair against a wall or on a mat in such a way that it will not slip. Place your palms on the seat of the chair, shoulder-width apart. Activate your abdomen by drawing your belly button in toward your spine. Step back, allowing your spine to lengthen and your head to come between your upper arms. Hold for 10 breaths, working your way up to a minute or two. (**3.33**)

2. When you are ready to release, step forward; bend your knees, keeping your spine long as you gracefully come to a standing position.

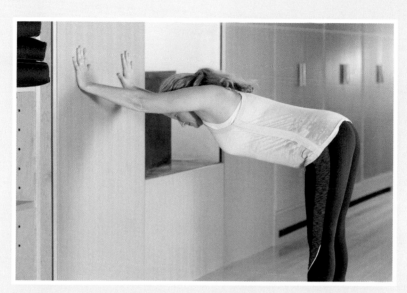

3.32 | Downward Facing Dog (variation 1)

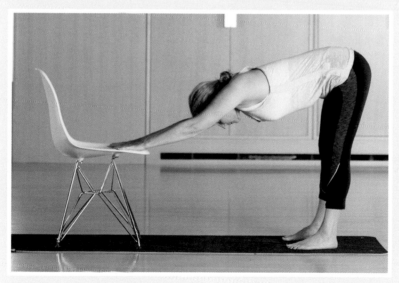

3.33 | Downward Facing Dog (variation 2)

COBRA
(belly down backbend)

Backbends provide much-needed opening of the chest and front body, which aids breathing and digestion. The floor supports and stabilizes as you lengthen the spine with the fluidity of a cobra. Don't do this posture if you are pregnant or have had recent abdominal surgery. If you have a "bad back," take this posture very slowly, lifting then lowering only slightly (if at all), as a breathing exercise.

1. Lie on the floor, belly down, with the legs together. If you can, let the big toes touch each other. Ground your lower body by pressing your hips and pelvis into the floor. Lightly engage the muscles of the legs, as though water were flowing through them toward the toes.

2. Place your hands under or behind (in the direction of your belly button) the shoulders, elbows pressing toward one another. Forehead or chin to the floor. (**3.34**)

3. Engage your buttock (butt) muscles and press the hips into the floor. Exhale, and on the inhale, lengthen through the crown of the head, roll the shoulders back and down, and slowly lift the head a few inches off the floor. Think about lengthening the spine, and extending along the spine evenly.

4. With each exhale, ground the base of the spine into the floor by pressing through the hips and reactivating the legs. With each inhale, open and lift the heart by expanding through the chest so that the collarbones float wider away from each other and the shoulders continue to release down the back. (**3.35**)

5. Keep your back relaxed. If you feel your back muscles grip or get tense, lower down, and once your back is fully relaxed, try the process of lifting into this backbend (beginning with step 3 above) while keeping your back soft.

(continued on pg. 60)

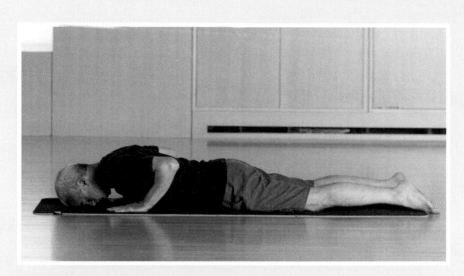

3.34 | Cobra

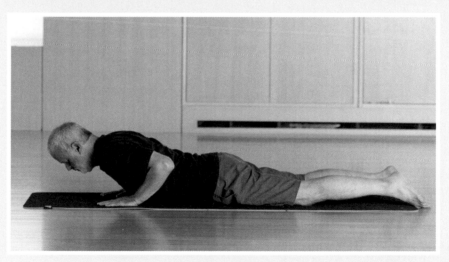

3.35 | Cobra

6. Practice coming to your fullest expression of this backbend for five to 10 breaths, building to 1 or 2 minutes. (**3.36**)

7. Inhale, and on the exhale, lower your head back to the floor, then release your arms.

8. Bend into the knees and let your feet slowly swing from side to side, to release and relax the lower back.

WORKING DEEPER

Another belly down backbend that further strengthens and lengthens is to:

- *Root the pelvis into the floor. Let your arms extend along the side of the body but a few inches away from your sides, palms down.*
- *Exhale, and on the inhale, lift the arms and the legs off the floor, lengthening through the crown of the head, reaching through arms and legs.*
- *You can do this as a breathing exercise, lifting on the inhale, and releasing back to the floor on the exhale. You can hold for several breaths at the top of the lift. If your back is strong, you can further deepen by extending the arms over your head for the longest position on the floor, arms reaching forward, feet reaching back.*

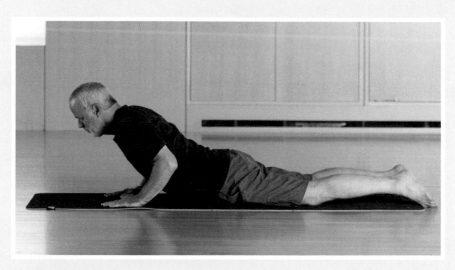

3.36 | Cobra

AWARENESS:

Backbends tend to be therapeutic for nearly everyone. They help create space in the chest allowing you to breathe more fully and have more energy. Most of us have very little awareness of what is happening behind our backs, and backbends remind us that we do have a back body. The beauty of belly down backbends is that they give us safety to explore these freeing postures.

SEATED FORWARD FOLD

Forward fold teaches lengthening and self-acceptance. The aim of this posture is not to get your head to the floor. Rather, keep the spine straight and cultivate space in your low back with patience and breath.

1. Sit up straight on the edge of a cushion or blanket with your legs out in front of you. Spread your toes to activate the feet, and let the muscles in your legs become active and hug to your bones. Root the hips and tailbone downward. Roll the shoulders back and down. (**3.37**)

2. Exhale, and then on the inhale, reach the arms up overhead. Relax the shoulders down the back. Gently engage the belly.

3. Inhale, lengthen upward through the crown of the head, then on an exhale, reach through the arms and hands as you gently bend at the hip, chest open, folding just an inch or two forward. Imagine someone has his/her hand on your lower back, gently pressing it forward so that it does not round.

4. Inhale, and on the exhale, release your arms and hands down to your legs or the floor. Keep the chest wide and open, shoulders rolled down the back, and continue to lengthen out the crown of your head. Lengthen on each inhale, and with the exhale, gently deepen the posture by releasing forward and accepting your back in whatever condition and degree of flexibility it is in. Avoid the temptation to press or push into this forward fold. Continue to lengthen through the crown of your head. Begin by holding this posture five to 10 breaths, and work up to 1 to 2 minutes. (**3.38, 3.39**)

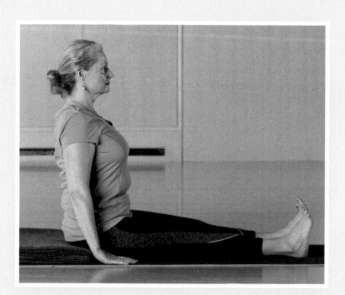

AWARENESS:

In a forward bend, lead with your open and wide chest. Accept that in this stretch, like all postures, you are right where you need to be to learn the lesson for which you are ready. Breathe and relax.

3.37 | Seated Forward Fold

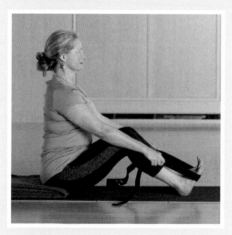

3.38 | Seated Forward Fold

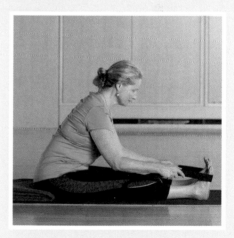

3.39 | Seated Forward Fold

SEATED SPINAL TWIST

Twists wring the effects of stress out of the spine. So, they may help relieve backaches, neck, shoulder and mental strain, and tension headaches. As you rotate into a twist, you press and move your kidneys and digestive system. This can improve digestion and reduce general sluggishness. Your spine and hips can become more flexible. Skip this posture if you have had an abdominal operation, or are suffering from a hernia, stomach, or abdominal problem. Practice twists while you are pregnant only under the guidance of a skilled instructor.

1. Come into a comfortable seated position, legs straight out in front of you. If your back is not comfortable as you sit on the floor, sit on a cushion or blanket. Tip your pelvis forward slightly, to help you achieve a straight spine.

2. Step your left leg over your right and keep your left foot on the floor and your left knee bent. (**3.40**)

3. Optional: Bend the right knee so that you can tuck your right foot alongside your left hip. If there is strain in the knee or hip, or the hip lifts off the floor, straighten the right leg.

4. Sit up straight, exhale, and on the inhale, let your left hand float up in front of you, straight arm, to shoulder height. Relax the shoulder down your back.

5. Inhale and lengthen up through the spine, and on the exhale, beginning at the base of the spine, gently twist to the right. Never push or force the twist; keep the neck and shoulders relaxed. With each inhale, lengthen up through the crown of the head. With each exhale, move until you reach a comfortable twist for you (you can still breathe deeply, there are no grabbing or straining feelings in the back). (**3.41**)

6. Hold the twist and breathe for 10 breaths, working up to 1 or 2 minutes in the posture.

7. Release the posture as slowly and deliberately as you entered it, slowly unwinding until you are in a seated position looking forward. Bring the left leg back next to the straight right leg. Smile.

8. Repeat, stepping the right leg over the left, and following the directions to gently twist to the left.

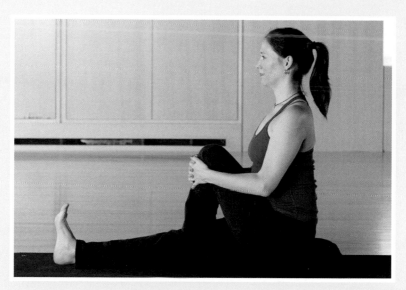

3.40 | Seated Spinal Twist

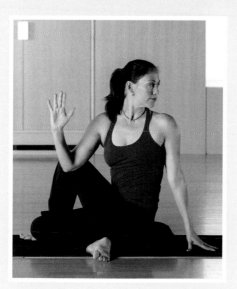

3.41 | Seated Spinal Twist

AWARENESS:

Only twist around a straight spine. If crossing your legs to look more like the yoga pictures causes one hip to lift and your spine to curve, please don't twist. Rather, keep one leg straight so as not to sacrifice this central alignment. Less is more in twists; keep your spinal twist soft. Let it be about relaxing rather than pressing or pushing. Our cervical spine (neck) is the most flexible part of the spine, but benefits the least from a deep twist. So, the mind might think it's doing well to rotate the neck deeply: Resist that temptation! Instead let the twist begin at the base of the spine, and be especially fluid in the neck.

COBBLER
(fold or squat with soles together)

This "bound angle" posture tones the lower torso, and creates space in the hips. It is thought to strengthen the bladder, aid menstrual issues, and is wonderful for pregnancy, particularly when done in the standing squat modification.

1. Sit comfortably on a cushion or blanket with your legs out in front of you. Sit up straight, with your hips rolling slightly forward so that the spine can be long. Engage the belly.

2. Draw the soles of the feet together, letting the knees drop out. If your knees do not reach to the floor, place a cushion or block under them. (**3.42**)

3. Inhale, lengthen up through the crown of the head, and on an exhale, fold forward with a straight spine over the legs. Take your time, and breathe into the stretch. Inhale and lengthen, and as you exhale, deepen the forward fold. (**3.43**)

4. Where can you relax? The groin? The jaw? Breathe and adjust for five breaths, working up to 1 minute.

5. Exhale, and on an inhale, come back up to seated. Slowly release the legs.

VARIATION: STANDING SQUAT

A variation of this posture is to squat, ultimately with your feet together (although that takes open hips; begin with feet apart, knees comfortable). Use the wall as a prop. (**3.44**)

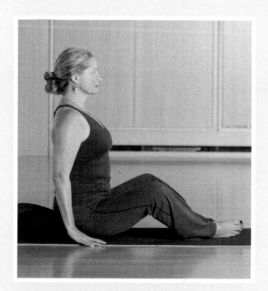

3.42 | Cobbler

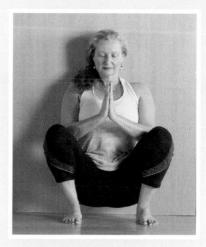

3.44 | Cobbler (variation)

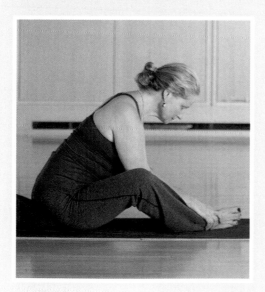

3.43 | Cobbler

AWARENESS:

Listen to your knees in this posture. If they hurt, release the posture, or practice it more gently by not worrying about getting your feet to touch one another. If your knees do not automatically drop to the floor, it simply means your hips are tight. Place pillows or a blanket under your knees so that your legs and the area around your hips can be relaxed. Like other forward folds, there is no prize for getting your head to the floor. Instead, breathe and focus on lengthening the body and gently opening your hips.

HERO
(kneeling foot stretch)

In yoga, your feet are considered the doors of the gate to your temple (if your temple is your body). Hero is an excellent posture for stretching the feet.

1. Begin on your knees, body upright. If this is uncomfortable, use cushions, blankets, and other props to support you. Align your hips with your knees, and your feet with the hips.

2. Roll your toes under. Big toes touching if possible. If not, keep the feet parallel. (**3.45, 3.46**)

3. Inhale, and on the exhale, sit back onto the heels. Breathe and relax for five breaths.

4. Inhale and lift the hips off the feet and on the exhale, roll the toes so that the tops of the feet are on the floor (soles of feet upward), heels together.

5. Inhale, and on the exhale, sit back onto the heels. Lift your abdomen and spine as your hips drop down, head lifts up. Breathe and relax for five breaths.

6. On an exhale, lower the hips toward the floor as the heels move apart from one another to make room for your buttocks. If you feel sensation in your knees, raise your hips higher or release.

7. To release, come back to your knees.

WORKING DEEPER
You can move back and forth between toes under and back as a flow with your breathing to open and stretch the feet.

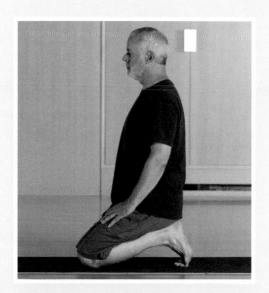

3.45 | Hero

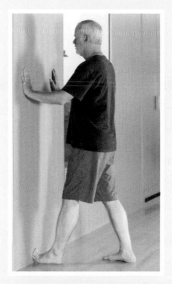

3.47 | Hero (variation)

AWARENESS:
Be kind to your knees in this posture with props (like a blanket under them). You can also place a towel behind the knees for more space, or use cushions to get the hips higher. This one may be uncomfortable, but take it slow for a gentle stretch that can be good medicine for stretching the feet. If this posture is too uncomfortable, you can get a similar stretch standing and against a wall. If you have diabetic neuropathy, do not do this posture. **(3.47)**

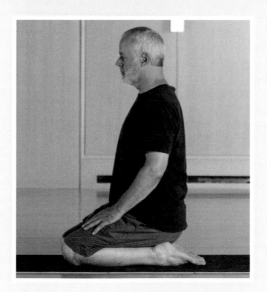

3.46 | Hero

BRIDGE
(backbend on the floor)

This stable backbend on the floor allows for a relaxed neck and shoulder alignment as you expand the chest and lengthen the front body. The spine is a bridge between your shoulders and feet, which stay firmly on the floor.

1. Lie on your mat, knees bent and in line with your feet. Place your feet under your knees. Draw your elbows along the sides of your body. Roll your shoulders down the back and release them toward the floor, so that the chest is wide and open. (**3.48**)

2. Press into the elbows and the feet. Exhale, and on the inhale, let the chest expand, and that movement lifts your spine off the floor. (**3.49**)

3. With each inhale, let your breath lift you higher, hips pressing up, buttocks slightly engaged, knees hip distance apart. With each exhale, soften and relax while holding the structure of the posture.

4. Let the elbows walk toward one another a bit behind the back to continue to open the chest. If it's comfortable, clasp your hands behind the back, keeping your elbows pressing into the floor.

5. Reach the hips up and away toward the knees. Continue to root down through the feet and elbows, and open the chest.

6. Breathe in this posture for 10 breaths, keeping the back relaxed. Work your way up to 1–2 minutes in the posture.

7. Inhale, and on the exhale, slowly release, vertebra by vertebra, back to the floor. Relax and release. Straighten the legs.

HEALTHY SPINE, HEALTHY BODY
Appreciation of the benefits of a flexible body is part of why yoga is so popular. The spine is the central structure of your whole body, so having flexibility and strength around your spine is one of the great gifts that yoga gives you.

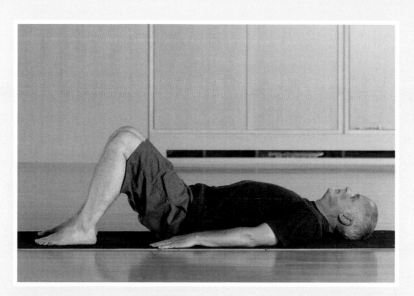

3.48 | Bridge

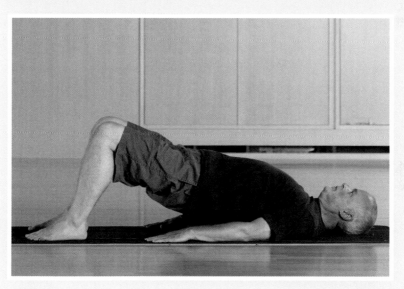

3.49 | Bridge

ABDOMINALS
(stand/walk on the ceiling and reclining twist)

Don't skip your abdominals! These postures strengthen your core—the muscular center of your body. When your core is strong, digestion improves, and your posture and energy level tend to improve.

VARIATION 1: STAND/WALK ON THE CEILING

1. Lie down face up. Hug your knees into your chest. Rock back and forth with your breath to release and warm up the lower back.

2. Place your hands along the sides of your body or under your buttocks to protect the lower back; engage the belly.

3. Press the soles of your feet up as if you were going to stand on the ceiling. Keep your shoulders melting into the floor. If you feel this in the low back, bend the knees a bit. This is your standing on the ceiling posture. Breathe and hold for five to 10 breaths, working your way up to 1–2 minutes. (**3.50**)

4. Keep rooting the hips into the floor, and do the work of the posture from the abdominal muscles, not the back.

5. Inhale, and on the exhale, slowly lower the right leg down toward (without releasing onto the floor). Keep the left leg lifted and left foot pressing up as though you were standing on the ceiling. Bend the knees if you feel twinges in the back, and take breaks, hugging the knees into the chest, when you need to. (**3.51**)

WORKING DEEPER
*To work the abdominals more deeply, lift your chest and shoulders up toward the sky. Resist reaching with the chin. Rather, keep the chin tucked and neck relaxed. (**3.52**)*

(continued on pg. 74)

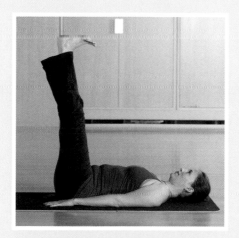

3.50 | Abdominals (variation 1)

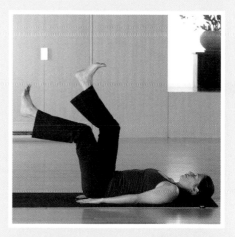

3.51 | Abdominals (variation 1)

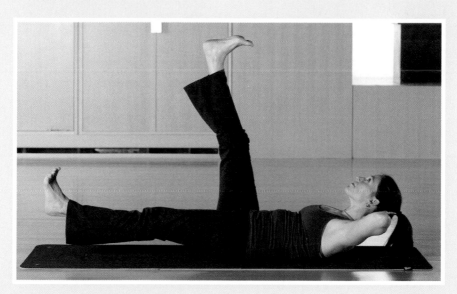

3.52 | Abdominals (variation 1)

6. Inhale, and on the exhale, slowly lower the left leg down toward the floor, and the right leg lifts back up as though the right foot were to stand on the ceiling.

7. Hug the knees into the chest, and gently roll the hips to release and breathe into the lower back. Begin with five on each side, and work your way up to 7–10 minutes of abdominals.

VARIATION 2: RECLINING TWIST

1. Hug the knees to the chest. Bring the arms out to a T position, palms facing down. Shift the hips about an inch to the left.

2. Engage the belly, and lift your legs so that the knees are over the hips, knees bent to 90 degrees. (**3.53**)

3. Inhale, and on the exhale, slowly and with control, lower your knees to the right until they hover over the floor. Rotate your engaged belly to the left. Take three long breaths. (**3.54**)

4. Draw your knees into your chest and roll to center. Repeat on the second side. Begin with three of these on each side and work up to your full 7–10 (or more!) minutes of abdominals. (**3.55**)

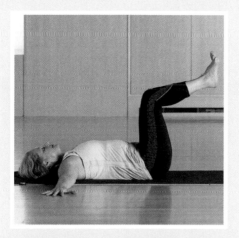

3.53 | Abdominals (variation 2)

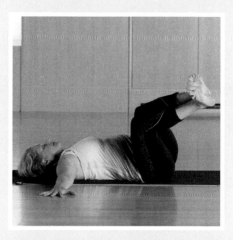

3.54 | Abdominals (variation 2)

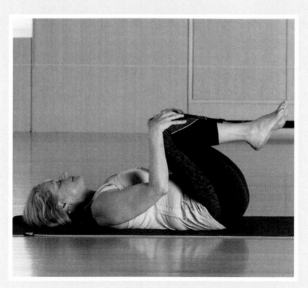

3.55 | Abdominals (variation 2)

AWARENESS:

Let's talk belly anatomy. There are a number of muscles in the abdomen. One long muscle runs up the center of your torso, and a variety of oblique muscles wrap around you. This matrix of muscle can be strengthened and toned. A strong core stabilizes the back and improves digestion and overall function, so it is worth the effort. The instruction to engage the belly means to activate the muscular matrix of the abdomen. To do this, think of each muscle hugging in toward the spine.

WIND-RELIEVING

Yes, this posture can help you pass gas, and it also opens the hips and gently massages the belly and digestive organs.

1. Lie down face up. Bend your right knee and take your right shin with both hands. Intertwine your fingers for a stronger grip.

2. Inhale, and on the exhale, roll the shoulders down the back, draw the elbows alongside your body, and breathe as you imagine breathing space into your right hip socket.

3. With each inhale create space in the hip, with each exhale relax around the hip joint as you engage the arms to deepen the stretch in the hip and massage the right torso. (**3.56**)

4. Hold and work the posture for five breaths. Release back to both legs straight. Repeat on second side. Relax. Begin with three repeats, and work your way up to three repeats of 10 breaths.

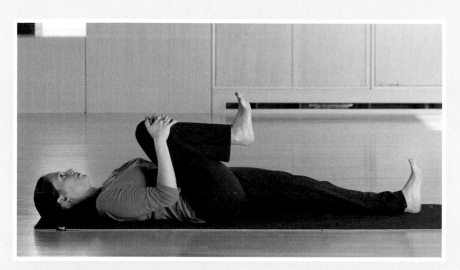

3.56 | Wind-relieving

LEGS UP THE WALL
(supported inversion)

Inversions are some of the most therapeutic postures in yoga, but they can be hard to get in and out of safely. This posture eases you into an inversion practice, and lets your hips and shoulders, rather than your more delicate neck, bear your weight. Getting upside down is thought to support all the cleansing aspects of our physiology. It also changes your usual point of view. Do not do this posture if you have diabetic retinopathy, glaucoma, high blood pressure, or recent back surgery. If you are pregnant, do inversions only under the guidance of a skilled teacher.

1. Sit on the floor against the wall, with one hip on the wall. (**3.57**)

2. Inhale, engage the belly, and on the exhale, swing your legs up the wall as you swing your torso to the floor. (**3.58**)

3. Get comfortable, shimmying the hips closer to the wall. If it feels better to keep the knees bent, do that.

4. Check your alignment: You want your nose in alignment with your belly button, right between the hips, right between the knees, and right between the big toes. Imagine a plumb line dropping down into a point between your eyebrows, and anchoring the back of your head to the floor. Imagine the chin and forehead in the same place (so the head is centered). The curve in the neck is there, and the neck is relaxed.

5. Stay here for five to 10 breaths, exhaling deeply, and letting the inhale flow in on its own. With each exhale, imagine tension flowing away from within your body.

6. To release, bend your knees and roll to the side.

WORKING DEEPER

- *Use your yoga block. Bend your knees to press your feet into the wall, press down through your elbows, and lift your hips off the wall. Keep the neck relaxed. Place the block at a comfortable level under the hips. You're there! Imagine walking the elbows toward one another behind the back to open the chest. Breathe and relax. (**3.59**)*

- *To further deepen, use the taller levels of the block. Hold this posture for five to 10 breaths, and work your way up to 10 minutes.*

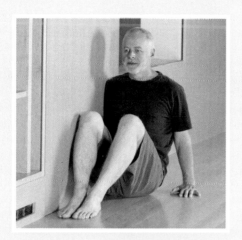

3.57 | Legs up the wall

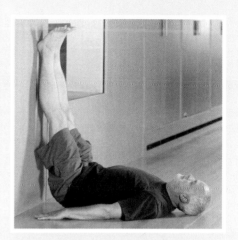

3.58 | Legs up the wall

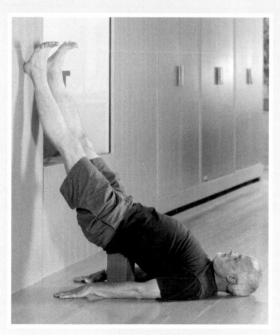

3.59 | Legs up the wall

AWARENESS:

Getting upside down so that your lungs are higher than the heart facilitates your exhale. If your inversion gets to the point where you are this far upside down, take advantage of the situation by exhaling deeply. When your digestive system is higher than your lungs (not your usual position!), your digestive organs get a gentle massage from the movement of your lungs as you breathe. When your legs are reaching up the wall, it facilitates their blood flow. Remember not to do inversion postures if you have diabetic retinopathy, glaucoma, or high blood pressure.

CORPSE POSE
(relaxation and integration)

The deep relaxation of yogic sleep allows you to receive the gifts of your practice. This is your sweet reward, so let it be delicious!

1. Prepare to lie on the floor (or in a bed if that works better for you). Gather props that will support you letting go into deep relaxation, perhaps a rolled blanket under the knees for space in the low back, or a small pillow under your head or neck. Soft music may be helpful.

2. Put your socks on, as your body will cool down as you relax. You might enjoy a light blanket over your body.

3. Once you are settled, take three breaths to engage all the muscles; scrunch up your face, makes fists, engage your buttocks—tight, then exhale and release with an "ahhh." Do this two more times.

4. Align the body for relaxation. Roll your hands up toward the ceiling, and let the legs relax. Let your back body become soft and release into the floor, front body relaxed, head, scalp, and face release.

Neck relaxes, chest relaxes, arms relax, belly relaxes, legs relax, feet, ankles, and toes relax.

5. In your mind's eye, see yourself receiving the gifts of your practice. See and feel your body stronger, lighter, and more flexible. See and feel the organs of your body supporting you by processing the good food you give yourself.

6. You are awake and alert, but relaxing. While sleeping is generally good, should you fall asleep during this exercise you are no longer practicing. If you find yourself dosing or your mind wandering off, bring your attention back to focus on your breathing. (**3.60**)

7. Begin with a few minutes of relaxing, perhaps to quiet music or a relaxation CD. You can practice this posture for 10–20 minutes per day.

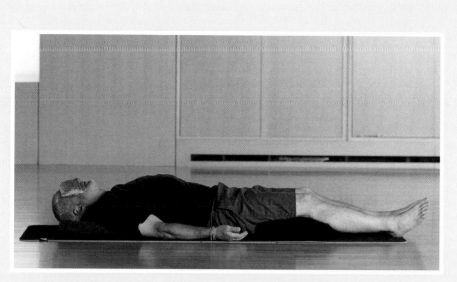

3.60 | Corpse

Chapter 4
Programs for Every Body

*It is helpful to realize that this very body
that we have, sitting right here right now...
with its aches and its pleasures...
is exactly what we need to be fully human,
fully awake, fully alive.*

— PEMA CHÖDRÖN

It is one thing to know a few yoga postures and breathing techniques. Weaving postures together into flows or programs is how your practice comes to life. Placing postures into a well-designed program is an art and science in itself. This is how you customize a yoga practice to meet your personal health needs and fitness goals.

In this chapter, you will find a variety of short and longer programs ranging from gentle to moderate to more vigorous. If you are new to yoga, begin with the gentle short programs and practice daily, if possible. As you become comfortable with the postures and flow of the short programs, slowly increasing the length and pace of your practice to add more vigor may improve your level of fitness. You can also try holding postures a little longer to improve your strength and stamina.

As your skill and comfort increase, move on to the moderate or more vigorous programs. Move from the short to the longer programs, and monitor yourself for changes. As you increase the pace of your practice, be sure to check your blood sugar when you finish, to make sure that you are not experiencing low blood sugars. Remember that exercise uses glucose and over time increases insulin sensitivity, so that you may need to make changes in your medications, especially if you are taking insulin (see Chapter 2 for more information)

Also, it is important to remember that with any new form of exercise, it is best to consult with your medical provider before beginning your practice. He or she can help you adapt your practice to support your individual health needs.

Most yoga teachers agree that when you are first starting your practice, it is better to do a little every day, rather than one long session once a week. Daily practice reinforces the habit of exercise, and makes it more likely to become a regular part of your routine.

A full yoga program usually consists of a centering posture or breathing exercise to start your practice; a series of more active postures designed to stretch and strengthen the entire body; and a relaxation to end your practice. The purpose of beginning and ending with relaxing or centering postures is to take the time to bring your mind, breath, and body into the same place. Avoid the tenden-

STRETCH VS. STRAIN

Learning to tell the difference between the sensations of stretch and overstretch or strain is key. They feel different in your body. Over time if you pay attention you will recognize the difference between a helpful stretch and an unhelpful overstretch or strain. Your experience will enable you to stretch at the edge of your comfort and increase your flexibility without dropping over the edge into overstretching.

Here are some physical signs that can help you tell the difference between stretch and overstretch:

STRETCH	OVERSTRETCH OR STRAIN
Feels comfortable.	Is not comfortable.
It is easy to breathe in a relaxed way.	Breath gets sharper, more ragged or strained.
Your face stays relaxed.	You notice strain or a grimace on your face, or your jaw is tense.
The sensation in the muscle is warm and pleasant and you can relax and breathe into it.	Sensation in the muscle is hot and unpleasant and it is difficult to focus on breathing. It is difficult to relax.

cy to rush through your practice. Remember that one of the goals of yoga is to reduce stress, which tends to make healthy lifestyle choices easier. Taking the time to center and relax your mind and body before starting your program will help you cultivate a sense of calm in your yoga practice and daily life.

Short Programs

Use these short programs to ease fully into your new yoga home practice. They can also be helpful when time is tight but you want to practice. The programs include specific postures that are described in Chapter 3.

If you have complications of diabetes or other medical conditions, review the modifications suggested in Chapter 2 (pg. 23), and in this chapter, before you begin.

If you are just beginning yoga and have type 1 or type 2 diabetes, alternating programs 1, 2, and 3 for the first week will provide you a gentle introduction to yoga breathing, gentle movement, and relaxation. Then, begin to move into longer or more moderate or vigorous practice as you are able and would like. Alternatively, stay with and enjoy short programs.

PROGRAM 1 ▶
10 minutes | gentle
This program gently explores movement and tone in your torso, the core of your body surrounding many organs, and balance. Use modifications of postures described in Chapter 3 if you feel unsteady.

Begin seated. Center yourself, then do belly breath followed by wave-sounding breath for 2 minutes or longer.

Move to standing position. Continue wave-sounding breath as you practice mountain, half moon, tree, seated spinal twist, bridge, and relaxation in corpse.

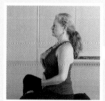
Belly breath (pg. 14)

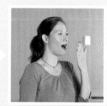
Wave-sounding breath (pg. 16)

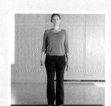
Mountain (pg. 34)

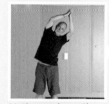
Half moon (pg. 36)

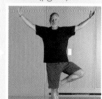
Tree (pg. 44)

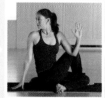
Seated spinal twist (pg. 64)

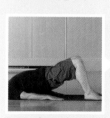
Bridge (pg. 70)

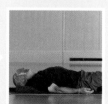
Corpse (pg. 80)

PROGRAM 2 ▶
10 minutes | gentle

This is a quiet program to enhance rest and relieve tension. Let this program be an exploration of your breath and movement.

Begin lying down on your back. Relax in corpse. Then belly breath lying down; wave-sounding breath lying down. Then roll onto your belly and practice cobra as a breathing exercise by lifting with the inhale, and lowering with the exhale. Finish with the child pose; cat and dog; child again; and relaxation in corpse.

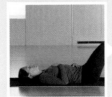
Belly breathing in corpse (pg. 14)

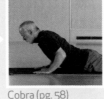
Cobra (pg. 58)

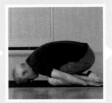
Child (pg. 32)

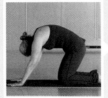
Cat and dog (pg. 30)

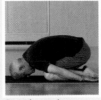
Child (pg. 32)

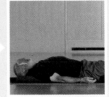
Corpse (pg. 80)

PROGRAM 3 ▶
10 minutes | gentle

This program can be helpful for people with insomnia. As you practice, clear the mind, perhaps with an image of packing thoughts into a box that you may reopen tomorrow. Focus on sensations in your body, and as distracting thoughts arise, pack them away. Return your attention to the present moment and follow the course of your inhale and exhale. Imagine relaxing your mind as you would relax a muscle.

Begin seated. Do an easy belly breath followed by the alternate nostril breath for 3 minutes or longer. Then do the hero pose; legs up the wall; seated forward fold; and finally, relaxation in corpse.

Belly breath (pg. 14)

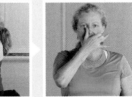
Alternate nostril (pg. 18)

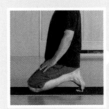
Hero (pg. 68)

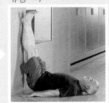
Legs up the wall (pg. 78)

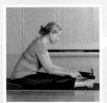
Seated forward fold (pg. 62)

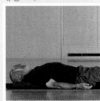
Corpse (pg. 80)

PROGRAM 4 ▶

10–15 minutes | gentle to moderate

This program is designed specifically for people with low back pain, but it is also helpful for keeping your spine flexible. Work gently and slowly. When you do this for the first time, you may choose to do just one of the abdominal strengtheners, and build up to doing both over time. As you move, focus on creating ease and space in the low back and wherever you feel discomfort. Imagine your breath filling your back body with relaxed comfort.

Lie down on your back, bend your knees, and place your hands on your knees, fingers pointing toward toes. With the inhale, straighten your arms and let the knees release away, and on the exhale, bend your arms to squeeze the knees toward the chest. With each inhale, notice the back lift slightly off the floor, and press into the floor with the exhale. Continue this breath for several minutes, then practice wave-sounding breath (pg. 16) as you do the wind relieving pose.

For abdominal postures (make sure to place hands under buttocks): Begin with the stand and walk on ceiling pose in the knees bent variation, taking frequent breaks, and then move into the knees to side variation; followed by bridge (gently lift and lower the hips as a breathing exercise). Can you feel each vertebra peel away then re-land on the floor as though you were lifting and lowering a string of pearls (pg. 70)? Finish with relaxation in corpse.

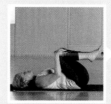

Wind relieving
(pg. 76)

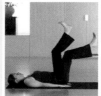
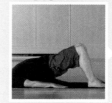

Stand/walk on the
ceiling (pg. 72)

Reclining twist (pg.
74)

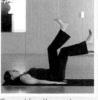
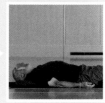

Bridge (pg. 70)

Corpse (pg. 80)

PROGRAM 5 ▶

10 minutes | gentle to moderate

This program includes postures that build overall strength and flexibility. Use modifications from Chapter 3 to keep your practice easy and comfortable.

Begin standing. Center yourself, and do a belly breath (pg. 14), followed by alternate nostril breath. Pause your breathing for just a second at the top of the inhale (holding in), and at the bottom of the exhale (holding out).

Follow this with the following poses: mountain; triangle; warrior 1; warrior 3; extended side angle (remember to do both sides of each posture); standing forward fold; bridge; legs up the wall. Finish with relaxation in cobra.

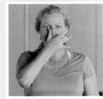
Alternate nostril (pg. 18)

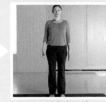
Mountain (pg. 34)

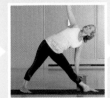
Triangle (pg. 42)

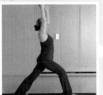
Warrior 1 (pg. 46)

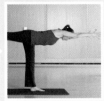
Warrior 3 (pg. 48)

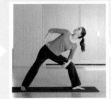
Extended side angle (pg. 52)

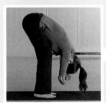
Standing forward fold (pg. 38)

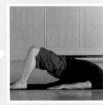
Bridge (pg. 70)

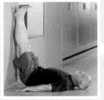
Legs up the wall (pg. 78)

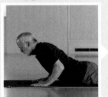
Cobra (pg. 58)

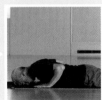
Relaxation in cobra (pg. 58)

PROGRAM 6 ▶

10 minutes | moderate

This program builds strength and balance. Remember to modify, use props, or balance against a wall if helpful.

Begin seated. Center yourself, and do belly breath followed by wave-sounding breath for 2 minutes or longer. Begin to pause for a second or two at the top of the inhale and at the bottom of the exhale.

Move mindfully to a standing position. Continue the wave-sounding breath, and then practice mountain; tree; warrior 1; warrior 2; warrior 3; standing forward fold; downward dog; bridge; and finally, relaxation in corpse.

Belly breath (pg. 14)

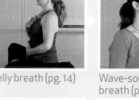
Wave-sounding breath (pg. 16)

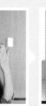

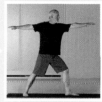
Mountain (pg. 34)

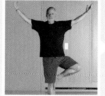

Tree (pg. 44)

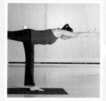
Warrior 1 (pg. 46)

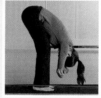
Warrior 2 (pg. 50)

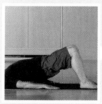
Warrior 3 (pg. 48)

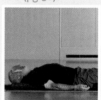
Standing forward fold (pg. 38)

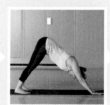
Downward dog (pg. 54)

Bridge (pg. 70)

Corpse (pg. 80)

PROGRAM 7 ▶

10 minutes | moderate

A practice to enhance your energy level.

Begin seated. Practice alternate nostril breathing with gentle holding for a second or two at the top of each inhale and at the bottom of each exhale. Do this for 3 minutes or longer.

Then move into the following poses: Table; cat and dog warm up; downward facing dog; standing forward fold; mountain; half moon; warrior 1; and warrior 2.

Move slowly between these two postures: inhaling into cobra and exhaling back to child, five times; then do bridge; legs up the wall; and finally, relaxation in corpse.

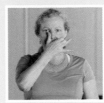
Alternate nostril (pg. 18)

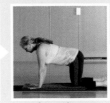
Table (pg. 28)

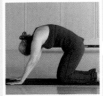
Cat and dog (pg. 30)

Downward dog (pg. 54)

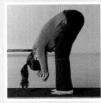
Standing forward fold (pg. 38)

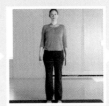
Mountain (pg. 34)

Half moon (pg. 36)

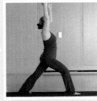
Warrior 1 (pg. 46)

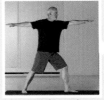
Warrior 2 (pg. 50)

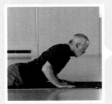
Cobra (pg. 58)

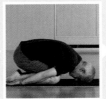
Child (pg. 32)

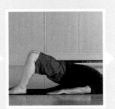
Bridge (pg. 70)

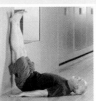
Legs up the wall (pg. 78)

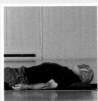
Corpse (pg. 80)

PROGRAM 8 ▶

10 minutes | moderate to vigorous

All of the programs can be helpful for managing stress. Here is one that will also build abdominal strength.

Begin seated. Alternate nostril breath with a holding of your breath in for a second or two at the top of your inhale, and holding your breath out for a second or two at the bottom of your exhale. Do this for 3 minutes or more.

Then do table posture; downward facing dog; and child. You will move between these three postures with each exhale for five repeats.

Then move into mountain; triangle; abdominals; bridge; legs up the wall; and finally, relaxation in corpse.

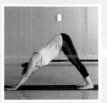
Alternate nostril (pg. 18)

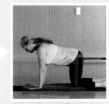
Table (pg. 28)

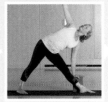
Downward dog (pg. 54)

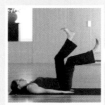
Child (pg. 32)

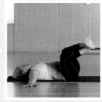
Mountain (pg. 34)

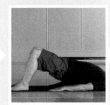
Triangle (pg. 42)

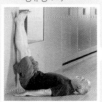
Stand/walk on the ceiling (pg. 72)

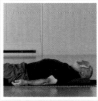
Reclining twist (pg. 74)

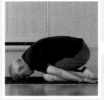
Bridge (pg. 70)

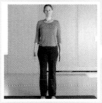
Legs up the wall (pg. 78)

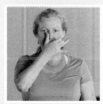
Corpse (pg. 80)

Longer Programs

The following programs are complete all-around practices. They include a full variety of postures: front and back bends, twists, and postures that focus on the major joints and muscle groups. Begin with the gentle programs and as you become proficient, explore the moderate programs, which may include a more active flow called "sun salutation."

PROGRAM 9 ▶
20 minutes | gentle

This program is designed for people with diabetes who have conditions that make getting up and down from the floor challenging, and who need to avoid inversions. This includes people with diabetic retinopathy, glaucoma, and high blood pressure.

Begin seated. Engage in belly breathing for at least 1 minute, then the wave-sounding breath for at least 1 minute. Alternate nostril breathing for 3 minutes or more.

Do a seated forward fold; seated spinal twist; cobbler; then lie down and do a gentle bridge, lifting and lowering just slightly. Follow with gentle abdominals with your hands under your buttocks and your knees bent. Finish with wind relieving; then stretch freely on the floor and move in the corpse position.

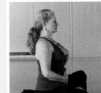
Belly breath (pg. 14)

Wave-sounding breath (pg. 16)

Alternate nostril (pg. 18)

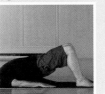
Seated forward fold (pg. 62)

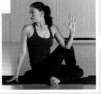
Seated spinal twist (pg. 64)

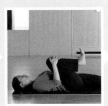
Cobbler (pg. 66)

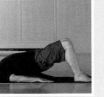
Bridge (pg. 70)

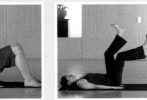
Abdominals (pg. 72)

Wind relieving (pg. 76)

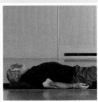
Corpse (pg. 80)

PROGRAM 10 ▶
30 minutes | gentle
A gentle and enjoyable all-around program to easefully build stamina.

Begin seated. Do wave-sounding breath for at least 1 minute, then add holding-the-breath at the top of the inhale and bottom of the exhale. Do alternate nostril breath; breathe and get centered for 5 minutes or more.

Move into mountain; half moon; tree; triangle; warrior 2; standing forward fold; child; seated spinal twist; cobbler; hero; wind relieving; bridge; legs up the wall; and finally, relaxation in corpse.

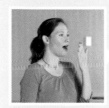
Wave-sounding breath (pg. 16)

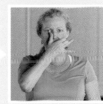
Alternate nostril (pg. 18)

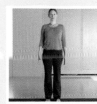
Mountain (pg. 34)

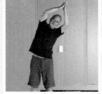
Half moon (pg. 36)

Tree (pg. 44)

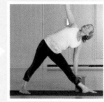
Triangle (pg. 42)

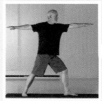
Warrior 2 (pg. 50)

Standing forward fold (pg. 38)

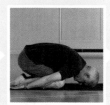
Child (pg. 32)

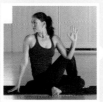
Seated spinal twist (pg. 64)

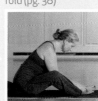
Cobbler (pg. 66)

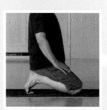
Hero (pg. 68)

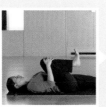
Wind relieving (pg. 76)

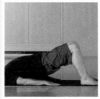
Bridge (pg. 70)

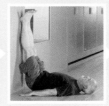
Legs up the wall (pg. 78)

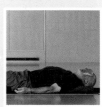
Corpse (pg. 80)

PROGRAM 11 ▶

30 minutes | gentle to moderate

This program is great when you are ready to step into a longer and more challenging practice. Take it at your own pace, and enjoy your strength, breath capacity, and flexibility.

Begin seated, and center yourself. Take an easy belly breath; wave-sounding breath; and alternative nostril breath, and repeat for 5 minutes or longer.

Move into child; cat and dog; mountain; half moon; triangle; warrior 1; downward facing dog; child for 10 to 12 breaths; then hero; seated spinal twist; abdominals, repeating two to five times with your knees bent; wind relieving; and finally, relaxation in corpse for 5 to 10 minutes. Then slowly come back to seated and sit quietly for a few minutes.

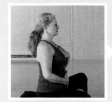
Belly breath (pg. 14)

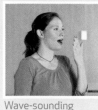
Wave-sounding breath (pg. 16)

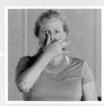
Alternate nostril (pg. 18)

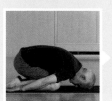
Child (pg. 32)

Cat and dog (pg. 30)

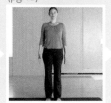
Mountain (pg. 34)

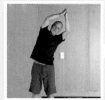
Half moon (pg. 36)

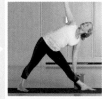
Triangle (pg. 42)

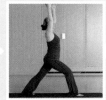
Warrior 1 (pg. 46)

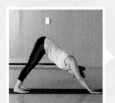
Downward dog (pg. 54)

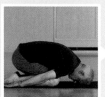
Child (pg. 32)

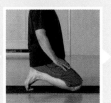
Hero (pg. 68)

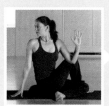
Seated spinal twist (pg. 64)

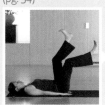
Abdominals (pg. 72)

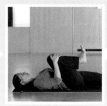
Wind relieving (pg. 76)

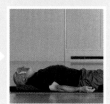
Corpse (pg. 80)

SALUTATION TO THE SUN ▶
version 1 | moderate

Sun salutation is a series of postures used in many yoga traditions as the heart of a flow (also called vinyasa) practice. In this flow, you move with the rhythm of your breath from posture to posture without pausing in between, and usually without staying in postures for longer than a few breaths. This tends to add vigor and heat to the practice. There are many variations of salutation to the sun. We are describing two versions; the first is more moderate and the second, more vigorous. Remember to support your back by keeping your knees slightly bent.

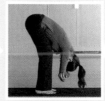
Mountain (pg. 34)

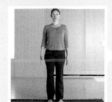
Standing forward fold (pg. 38)

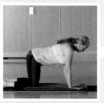
Table (pg. 28)

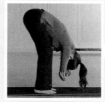
Cobra (pg. 58)

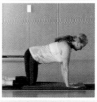
Table (pg. 28)

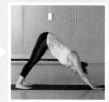
Downward dog (pg. 54)

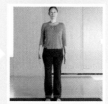
Standing forward fold (pg. 38)

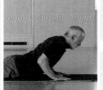
Mountain (pg. 34)

Exhale: Stand in mountain

Inhale: Mountain, arms overhead

Exhale: Dive forward with your belly engaged, knees slightly bent, to standing forward fold

Inhale: Come to a flat back

Exhale: Hands to the floor, come to table, then lower down onto your belly

Inhale: Cobra

Exhale: Lower to the floor

Inhale: Table

Exhale: Downward facing dog, knees bent); take five breaths in this posture

Inhale: Standing forward fold

Exhale: Stay in standing forward fold

Inhale: Mountain, arms overhead

Exhale: Mountain, arms at sides. Smile into your heart.

SALUTATION TO THE SUN ▶
version 2 | vigorous

Weaving this flow into your practice will create heat and strengthen your entire body. Work your way up to this version by taking several breaths to get from one posture to the next. Practice safe yoga alignment and take your time to prevent getting singed by the sun.

Exhale: Stand in mountain

Inhale: Mountain, arms overhead

Exhale: Standing forward fold

Inhale: Lower to the floor and into cobra

Exhale: Downward dog; stay for five breaths

Inhale: Warrior 1

Exhale: Lunge then lower to the floor

Inhale: Cobra

Exhale: Downward facing dog

Inhale: Step forward

Exhale: Standing forward fold

Inhale: Mountain, arms overhead

Exhale: Mountain, arms at side. Smile into your heart.

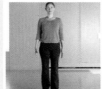
Mountain (pg. 34)

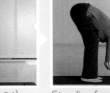
Standing forward fold (pg. 38)

Standing forward fold (pg. 40)

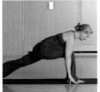
Cobra (pg. 58)

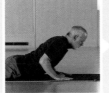
Downward dog (pg. 54)

Warrior 1 (pg. 46)

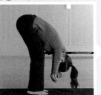
Warrior 1 lunge (pg. 48)

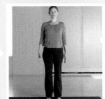
Cobra (pg. 58)

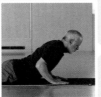
Downward dog (pg. 54)

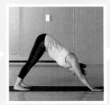
Standing forward fold (pg. 38)

Mountain (pg. 34)

PROGRAM 12 ▶

30–45 minutes | moderate to vigorous

Here is a practice centered on salutation to the sun. Notice how movement and breath work together in this flowing program; inhale lengthens, exhale softens and relaxes.

Begin seated, and center yourself. Take an alternate nostril breath with a moment of holding your breath at the top of your inhale and end of your exhale. Do the wave-sounding breath for 5 minutes or more.

Do child; table; downward facing dog, and hold here for 10 breaths or more. Step forward to standing forward fold. Then do the salutation to the sun, version 1; warrior 1; warrior 3; then, salutation to the sun, version 1; warrior 2; triangle; salutation to the sun, version 2; standing forward fold; cobra; child; seated spinal twist; salutation to the sun, version 1; cobbler; abdominals; salutation to the sun, version 1; bridge; legs up the wall; and finally, relaxation in corpse.

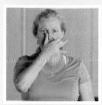
Alternate nostril (pg. 18)

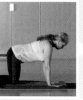
Wave-sounding breath (pg. 16)

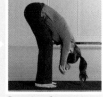
Child (pg. 32)

Table (pg. 28)

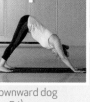
Downward dog (pg. 54)

Standing forward fold (pg. 38)

SALUTATION TO THE SUN
version 1

pg. 95

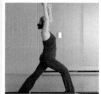
Warrior 1 (pg. 46)

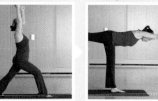
Warrior 3 (pg. 48)

SALUTATION TO THE SUN
version 1

pg. 95

Warrior 2 (pg. 50)

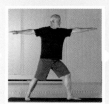
Triangle (pg. 42)

SALUTATION TO THE SUN
version 2

pg. 96

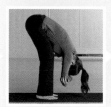
Standing forward fold (pg. 38)

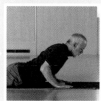
Cobra (pg. 58)

(continued on the next page)

(program 12 continued from previous page)

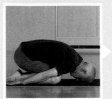

Child (pg. 32)

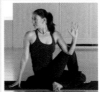

Seated spinal twist (pg. 64)

SALUTATION TO THE SUN version 1

pg. 95

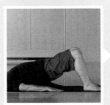

Cobbler (pg. 66)

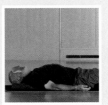

Abdominals (pg. 72)

SALUTATION TO THE SUN version 1

pg. 95

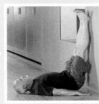

Bridge (pg. 70)

Legs up the wall (pg. 78)

Corpse (pg. 80)

PROGRAM 13 ▶

30–45 minutes | vigorous

Here is a more challenging program that builds strength, flexibility, breath capacity, and endurance. The key with a more physically demanding yoga practice is to keep a relaxed softness and ease in your breath, and to resist the temptation to push yourself. If your breath gets choppy or you find yourself pushing too hard, rest, relax, and come back to it. No rush.

Begin seated, and center yourself. Do an alternate nostril breath with wave-sounding breath for 5 minutes or more.

Move into child; table; downward facing dog, and hold for 10 breaths or more, then step forward to standing forward fold; salutation to the sun, version 2. Repeat three times, then move into warrior 1; warrior 3; salutation to the sun, version 2; warrior 2; triangle; salutation to the sun, version 2; standing forward fold; cobra; child; seated spinal twist; salutation to the sun, version 1; cobbler; abdominals; salutation to the sun, version 1; bridge; legs up the wall; and finally, relaxation in corpse.

Alternate nostril (pg. 18)

Wave-sounding breath (pg. 16)

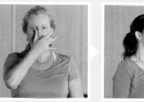
Child (pg. 32)

Table (pg. 28)

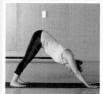
Downward dog (pg. 54)

Standing forward fold (pg. 38)

SALUTATION TO THE SUN version 2 (x3)

pg. 96

Warrior 1 (pg. 46)

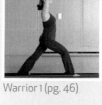
Warrior 3 (pg. 48)

SALUTATION TO THE SUN version 2

pg. 96

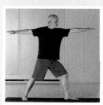
Warrior 2 (pg. 50)

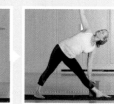
Triangle (pg. 42)

SALUTATION TO THE SUN version 2

pg. 96

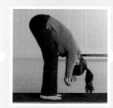
Standing forward fold (pg. 38)

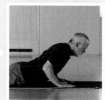
Cobra (pg. 58)

(continued on the next page)

(program 13 continued from previous page)

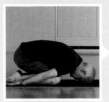

Child (pg. 32)

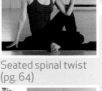

Seated spinal twist (pg. 64)

SALUTATION TO THE SUN version 1

pg. 95

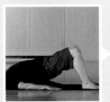

Cobbler (pg. 66)

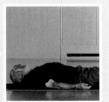

Abdominals (pg. 72)

SALUTATION TO THE SUN version 1

pg. 95

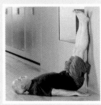

Bridge (pg. 70)

Legs up the wall (pg. 78)

Corpse (pg. 80)

Practices and Modifications for Pregnancy and Other Health Conditions

Just about everyone needs to modify some aspect of his or her yoga practice from time to time to accommodate aches and pains as well as ongoing medical conditions. Some health conditions, such as excess weight or just feeling out of shape, may make it difficult to hold certain postures due to discomfort or lack of strength. In these cases, the modifications discussed in Chapters 2 and 3 that involve using a chair, prop, or wall for support may be helpful. You may find that with increased practice you are able to perform the postures with increased comfort, ease, and confidence.

With some complications, however, it is better to avoid certain postures altogether. For instance, poses that increase blood flow to the head, such as downward dog or standing forward fold, may be unsafe for people with certain medical conditions and diabetes complications. The following recommendations will help you determine the modifications you may need if you have a diabetes-related complication. If you have questions or concerns about the safety of any of the poses presented in this chapter and your individual health conditions or diabetes complications, please speak with your health-care provider to make sure they are safe and appropriate for you.

Modifications for people with peripheral neuropathy or peripheral vascular disease

Wear socks and comfortable shoes. Keep your practice space clean and clear of anything that could cause injury to your feet. If standing poses are too uncomfortable, focus on seated or supine poses such as table, seated forward fold, or bridge, for example. Almost any standing pose can be modified

and done while seated in a chair or even lying down on the floor or in bed. Can you get creative with how you get the stretch and relaxation of yoga and take excellent care of yourself too?

Below is a modified short program that you might find helpful.

Modifications for people with diabetic retinopathy, glaucoma, or high blood pressure

Inversion postures, such as standing forward folds and downward dog, place the head below the heart, thereby increasing the amount of pressure in the head and

PROGRAM 14 ▶

10 minutes | gentle
A program for people with peripheral neuropathy or peripheral vascular disease.

Begin seated. Take an easy belly breath followed by an alternate nostril breath for 3 minutes or longer.

Do a seated forward fold; seated spinal twist; bridge; legs up the wall; and finally, relaxation in corpse.

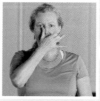
Belly breath (pg. 14)

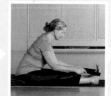
Alternate nostril (pg. 18)

Seated forward fold (pg. 62)

Seated spinal twist (pg. 64)

Bridge (pg. 70)

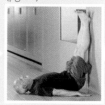
Legs up the wall (pg. 78)

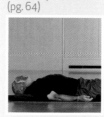
Corpse (pg. 80)

eyes. This is felt to be unsafe for people with diabetic proliferative retinopathy, glaucoma, or blood pressure that remains high (>140/90) despite medication. If you suffer from any of these conditions, it is best to avoid fully inverted postures.

You can, however, modify postures to be safer by keeping your head in line with your torso. For instance, try variation 1 of downward dog against the wall (pg. 56), making sure to keep your head in line with your torso.

If you have one of these conditions, the programs that are best for you to begin with are Programs 1, 2, 3, 4, 9, and 14. You can also try Programs 5, 10, and 11 with the modification to substitute variation 1 of downward dog (pg. 56) for the standing forward fold and downward dog in those programs.

Yoga during pregnancy

Yoga is a wonderful tool to improve health during and after pregnancy. Studies have found the practice of prenatal yoga to reduce depression, anxiety, and leg and back pain. Other studies have shown yoga to reduce the risk of preterm labor and low birth weight. Yoga has also been shown to reduce stress in high-risk pregnancies.

In recent years, it has become increasingly clear that fitness is important during and after pregnancy. In fact, exercise is an important tool to keep women who are diagnosed with diabetes during pregnancy (known as gestational diabetes) from developing type 2 diabetes later in life. While some women with gestational diabetes find their blood sugars return to normal after delivery, a large Canadian study found that nearly 19% of women previously diagnosed with gestational diabetes went on to develop type 2 diabetes within 9 years. In certain populations, this risk can be as high as 70%.

However, both observational and controlled studies have shown that regular exercise reduces this risk. In fact, women with gestational diabetes who engage in 150 minutes per week of moderate-intensity exercise after pregnancy can reduce their risk of developing type 2 diabetes by 47%.

For all of these reasons, yoga is an excellent form of gentle to moderate exercise during and after pregnancy. If you are just beginning your yoga practice, you may find it helpful to work with a qualified prenatal yoga teacher, to help you adapt your practice as your body changes from week to week.

The following programs are safe and gentle for women with gestational diabetes, and for women with type 1 or type 2 diabetes who are pregnant.

As you move through these programs, pay attention to how you feel and avoid strain or discomfort. Pay special attention to your hips, shoulders, wrists, and knee joints. Throughout the 2nd and 3rd trimesters of pregnancy, create a welcoming space for your baby by keeping your abdomen free, avoiding twists and forward folds.

PROGRAM 15 ▶

10 minutes | gentle

A program for pregnant women.

Begin seated. Do easy belly breaths for 6 minutes or longer.

Do the hero pose, moving between feet rolled under, then flat, with each exhale. Move to cobbler against the wall (stay as long as is comfortable) and then legs up the wall without a block (no height). Relax on your left side, with pillows under your knees and anywhere else that supports you, for 5 to 15 minutes.

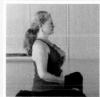
Belly breath (pg. 14)

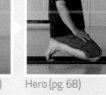
Hero (pg. 68)

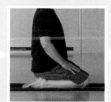
Hero (pg. 68)

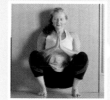
Cobbler (pg. 66)

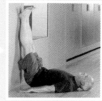
Legs up the wall (pg. 78)

PROGRAM 16 ▶

30 minutes | gentle

A program that gives the belly plenty of space, making it appropriate for pregnant women.

Begin seated. Do easy belly breaths and alternate nostril breaths for 10 minutes or longer.

Move to a standing position. Do mountain; tree; warrior 2; hero, moving between feet rolled under then flat with each exhale; cobbler against the wall (stay as long as is comfortable); and legs up the wall without a block (no height). Relax on your left side, pillows under your knees and anywhere else that supports you, for 5 to 15 minutes.

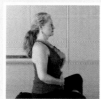
Belly breath (pg. 14)

Alternate nostril (pg. 18)

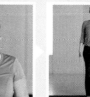
Mountain (pg. 34)

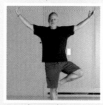
Tree (pg. 44)

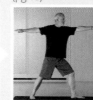
Warrior 2 (pg. 50)

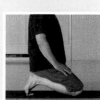
Hero (pg. 68)

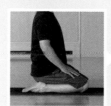
Hero (pg. 68)

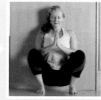
Cobbler (pg. 66)

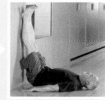
Legs up the wall (pg. 78)

INCREASED FLEXIBILITY DURING PREGNANCY

During pregnancy, the body produces a hormone called relaxin. This hormone makes ligaments more loose and flexible, which helps to open the pelvis during delivery. It can also increase the range of motion of other joints during pregnancy. Take care not to overstretch ligaments in the hips, wrists, or knees by not stretching more than a 90-degree angle during flexion (movement at the joint).

The Next Step

The programs in this book provide you a guide to begin and progress your yoga practice. Studying under the guidance of a skilled yoga teacher will also enhance and likely advance your practice. As you become more familiar with yoga breathing, postures, and programs, get curious about what is working for you, and creative with modifying your program to address your needs on a particular day. Chapter 5 will help you practice yoga not only on your yoga mat, but throughout your life.

Chapter 5
Yoga and Your Lifestyle

*To me, good health is more than just exercise
and diet. It's really a point of view and
a mental attitude you have about yourself.*

—JOHN F. KENNEDY

Everyone wants to be happy. We all want healthful lives. In our frenetic modern world, however, happiness can seem out of reach, especially if we are managing a health condition like diabetes. Living with and managing diabetes can at times challenge the most optimistic of us. Just how do you get from where you are to where you want to be?

The mental practice of yoga described in Chapter 2 can inform your entire lifestyle. Yoga's mental training can not only guide your physical practice, but can apply to all areas of managing your diabetes, including what, when, and how you eat, how well you manage your diabetes medications, your habits of rest and sleep, and even your personal and social relationships. Each of these aspects of your life may impact your ability to manage your diabetes. Yoga, mindfulness, and meditation may help people with diabetes make healthier choices. It's all about the power of pause.

Mindfulness:
The Power of Pause

Mindfulness is a type of meditation wherein you pay close attention to what is happening, moment by moment. You are not on autopilot. When you are mindful, you also adopt an attitude of nonjudgmental awareness. That is, it's not good, it's not bad, it just is. Nothing is better than anything else. Think of mindfulness as applying the mental practice of yoga to your daily life. Science has shown that mindfulness can be part of an effective approach to making lifestyle choices that can help you cope with and manage your diabetes.

Focused attention

Meditation is a process of quieting your physical body and mind. Yoga scholar Georg Feuerstein, PhD, described meditative absorption as a state of deep concentration in which your object of focus (examples include your breath, a sound, or the flame of a candle) takes your full attention.

Mindfulness is a type of meditation. In mindfulness, the object of focus is whatever you are experiencing. To practice you take a step back mentally, observing what is happening as if you were watching a good friend or beloved family member. In yoga this is often called witness consciousness. Have you ever had the experience that was so big—perhaps the first glimpse of your child or a scary storm—when you felt as though you were watching yourself from

across the room? Yogis might say that the person across the room is your witness—your observer. Rather than emotionally reacting, mindfulness offers a moment of pause to access the point of view of the observer within you.

The present moment

Have you ever noticed how your body reacts the moment you realize you have forgotten an appointment? You may feel a flush and tension in your jaw or neck. Noticing how emotions feel in your physical body can be a practice in mindfulness. As you practice, you are likely to notice ever more subtle messages. In mindfulness practice, you notice what is happening right now around you, inside your mind, and within your body. One way to practice is to become aware of each of your five senses: sight, touch, hearing, taste, and smell.

Nonjudgmental awareness

The Buddhist monk Thich Nhat Hanh writes beautifully about mindfulness. He describes doing the dishes mindfully, and washing a teapot as if it were a sacred object. It takes longer, he admits, but he is happy.

At the Kripalu Center for Yoga & Health, we use the term "compassionate self-observation" in many of our programs. The ability to see ourselves, our lives, and the choices we make with curiosity, compassion, and value is central to letting go of a critical mindset. That inner critic seems to prevent us from experimenting with change.

Mindfulness Meditations

Here is a collection of exercises that can support a mindful approach to managing your diabetes. Read through them, and begin with the one that most appeals to you. The more you practice, the more likely you are to experience the benefits of your effort.

Mindful of thoughts: Your internal dialogue

We all have automatic thoughts and beliefs. This exercise will help you to become more aware of your automatic thoughts, and provide a framework for looking at them and shifting them if you wish. Having negative, untrue, or unkind thoughts about yourself or others is completely normal. They are thoughts, and thoughts can be changed.

1. **Become aware of your internal dialogue.** Begin by noticing, as you go through your day, the things that you say to yourself. No need to do anything about it right now. Just notice. Get into the habit of noticing your thoughts. You might spend 1 day or 1 week just noticing before moving to the next step.

2. **Write it down.** Write down the things you say to yourself, particularly the things you say about yourself. Keep a running list of your self-talk. You might spend a week jotting down the things you say to yourself.

3. **Is it true? Is it helpful?** Look over the list of thoughts you came up with. Are there themes? If you are like most people, you have automatic thoughts that are rooted in beliefs you have had over much of your life. On page 108 is a list of common self-limiting thoughts. Do any of them sound familiar?

4. **Envision what you'd like your inner dialogue to sound like.** Reassuring? Loving? Just not so negative? Can you think of—then write down—a message or two that would be helpful for you to hear on a regular basis?

The more you practice this, the better you'll get at it. When you hear yourself judging someone else, reframe it. Give others the benefit of the doubt you wish you'd get. When you hear yourself complain about your life circumstances, remember one or two rays of light in your life. You can choose to focus on the light, or the dark.

Mindful attitude: Gratitude list

Making a list of the things you are grateful for is a simple practice that can change your perspective. Here are a few ideas to make it easy to count your blessings. Try one or more of these simple practices daily.

- In the car, on your way to or from work, think of five things that you are grateful for.

- Before you drift off to sleep, or when you first awake in the morning, do the same exercise. Think of five things that make you feel grateful.

COMMON SELF-LIMITING THOUGHTS

Always-or-never thoughts: *I never get a break; This always happens to me; Nobody cares about me.*

Dwelling on the negative and discounting the positive: *I had ice cream with family therefore I am weak and don't have any willpower; You only say that to be nice; It's no fun to be healthy; I know I can't do that.*

Emotional reasoning and "should" statements: *I feel inadequate therefore I am inadequate; I should eat better and exercise more.*

Labeling and blame: *He's a loser; She makes me feel bad, and then I eat; I'm too fat.*

For each self-limiting thought you notice, can you reframe it to be truer, positive, or reality-based? Below are some examples of how self-limiting thoughts might be reframed.

REFRAMING SELF-LIMITING THOUGHTS

Always-or-never thoughts are usually wrong. Reframe them with what is really true.

"*I never get a break*" can become, "*If something went wrong, there will be other opportunities.*"

"*People always take advantage of me,*" can become, "*I feel angry when you take advantage of me, but I know you can treat me fairly.*"

"*Nobody cares about me,*" can become, "*I feel lonely and frustrated right now.*"

Dwelling on the negative and discounting the positive tends to cultivate negative feelings and destructive action.

"*I had ice cream with family, therefore I failed and don't have any willpower,*" can become, "*I made a decision to eat ice cream and I enjoyed every bite!*"

"*You only say that to be nice,*" can become, "*Thank you for the compliment!*"

"*I can't have fun and be healthy,*" can become, "*I'll find fun in the healthy things I do.*"

"*I know I can't do that,*" can become, "*Nothing ventured, nothing gained...let me give it a try.*"

Reframe emotional reasoning and "should" statements with what is true.

"*I feel inadequate therefore I am inadequate,*" can become, "*I feel inadequate sometimes, but that doesn't mean I am inadequate.*"

"*I should eat better and exercise more,*" can become, "*I will feel better if I eat well and exercise more.*"

Labeling, personalization, and blame are at best distractions. Challenge these thoughts with kindness and truth.

"*He's a loser. I'm fat,*" can become, "*He goofed, but can do better. I'm having an issue with weight, but I can do something about it.*"

"*She makes me feel bad, then I eat,*" can become, "*I reacted to what she said, then ate instead of expressing my emotions in a healthier way. I can do better.*"

- Can't think of five things? How about three?

- What do you appreciate about yourself and your life? Make a list of your best traits, the good things that you have done for others, and the things you have done of which you are proud.

- Take every opportunity to notice the beauty in your day, be it a beautiful sky, the face of a family member, or things you encounter in your day. When you see beauty, pause to admire.

Yoga at the table: Mindful eating

Mindful eating is a powerful practice that can help you turn down the unhealthy messages you hear in the media and throughout the food environment, and tune into your internal guidance system with regard to what and how much to eat. Researchers Jean Kristeller, PhD, from Indiana State University and Ruth Wolever, PhD, from Duke University have conducted several studies with people with type 2 diabetes. In the studies, one group received training on the "Smart Choices" program for diabetes self-management. The other group learned one new skill: mindful eating.

At the end of 6 weeks, the outcomes for the two approaches were nearly the same. Both strategies did a good job of helping people manage their blood sugar. Imagine if you combine mindful eating with other ways you eat to manage your blood sugar? Why not try the experiment yourself?

Mindful Eating Meditation

Mindful eating makes you more aware of what and how much you eat and cultivates appreciation for your food. People tend to enjoy what they eat mindfully.

1. **Make a decision early in the day that you will eat mindfully during a meal.** Decide what it will be, and when you will do it. Give yourself 20 minutes for a snack, and longer for a simple meal.

2. **Prepare your food by hand, preferably without machines, in silence.** Choose a simple preparation such as peeling an orange or eating a slice of apple or simple salad. What can you make that nourishes your body? As you prepare your food, breathe, take your time, and slow down your movements. No rush. Appreciate each ingredient and each step of the process with all five senses. What do you notice about the color and texture? The aroma? Does it make a sound?

3. **Once prepared, sit down with your food in front of you.** Place both feet on the floor, and tune into the soft rhythm of your breath.

4. **When you are ready, begin to eat.** Take the time to appreciate each bite with all five senses. Chew slowly and completely. Can you chew each bite 20 times? 30? Enjoy the full flavor and variety of tastes and textures in each bite. Breathe and relax.

5. Once you complete your meal or snack in this way, pause and relax. This may be a good time to note your experience in a journal. What happened? What was challenging? Was it fun?

If you can't find the time to do this entire exercise, can you try taking one mindful bite at the next meal? Or, take three breaths before you begin to eat? What can you do to "chunk it down" so that the practice is doable in your life? You really can't do mindful eating incorrectly (although in front of the television is not a great idea). Just keep practicing.

Mindfulness and navigating change

You can practice a mindful approach to making a lifestyle change. Here is an exercise called "Create Your Mindful Lifestyle" that can guide you. In this exercise you set an intention for your work. When you set an intention, you clarify your motivation for action.

The steps outlined below will guide you in (1) remembering why you want to change; (2) identifying areas for experimentation; (3) using affirmations and setting realistic and achievable goals; and (4) developing an achievable plan of action and a system for learning from inevitable setbacks. This planning exercise can take a full hour, so feel free to do it over more than one sitting. Mindful eating and the other exercises can be helpful as tools to manage challenges you encounter.

1. **Set an intention.** Breathe, relax, and quiet your mind. What are you interested in bringing into your life through your efforts of managing your diabetes? (For example, "I want to manage my blood sugars.") How would you like to feel about it? Take a few minutes to write down your intention.

2. **Identify specific areas for experimentation.** Use the intention you set and information from your most recent self-monitoring and/or past experience to identify specific areas you'd like to shift. List three areas that are important to you. (Examples might include, "Checking blood sugars," "Eating more vegetables," or "Getting more exercise.")

1. _____

2. _____

3. _____

3. **Set a compassionate goal.** Select one area for experimentation from the list you made above. Answer all the questions that apply.

What is the experiment? What will you do?

Now get specific: How will you (or someone observing you) know that you are making progress?

- Specify a time period (e.g., week, month, vacation)
- Specify how often (e.g., daily, once a week)
- Specify how much (e.g., ½ cup, 1 oz., 30 min.)
- Specify where (e.g., home, restaurant, work)
- Specify with whom (e.g., family member, friends, co-workers)

4. **Develop affirmations.** These are clear statements of what you want to create that can support your goal. They are the fruit of your intention, and they actively bring intention into your daily life. Affirmations can be aspirational: They are a vision of what you intend to create.

Affirmations are:

- Written down
- Short, clear, and specific
- Stated in the present tense
- Stated in the positive
- Important to you personally
- Addressed to yourself (and include you); not about changing others

Write an affirmation that puts your intention into action. (For example: "I enjoy eating plenty of vegetables.")

5. **Develop a plan of action.** List the three challenges that you are most likely to encounter in your effort to reach your goal.

Challenge #1:

Challenge #2:

Challenge #3:

What will you do to manage your challenges in order to prevent them from derailing you?

To manage challenge #1, I will:

To manage challenge #2, I will:

To manage challenge #3, I will:

6. **Create a visualization.** The mental images we most frequently hold are what we create. Visualization will:

- Give you a strong positive feeling when you hold it
- Include you in the picture, doing your vision with fulfillment
- Be either literal or metaphoric
- Be written down and/or drawn as a picture

Visualize yourself practicing a behavior that will help you reach your goal. Write or draw your supportive visualization.

7. **Is it achievable?** How confident are you, on a scale of 0–100%, that you can reach this goal?

0%   25%   50%   75%   100%

If you are not at least 75% confident, modify your goal to increase the likelihood that you will be successful.

8. **Embody your affirmation.** Live it now. You create what you confidently expect. To germinate the mental seed, create a feeling of expectation and assumption that it is already happening for you, in you. What supports this feeling of certainty is:

A) *Daily repetition: Do the thing you want to do as often as you can remember to do it.*

B) *Walking your talk: Move, speak, and carry yourself as one who is this vision and has already achieved it.*

C) *Ongoing awareness and adjustment of your inner dialogue.*

9. **Seal the deal with a contract.** Write up an agreement with yourself. Here is one example:

I will begin working on the following goal and supporting affirmations:

On *(date)*, I will begin to self-monitor or journal to evaluate my progress in reaching my goal, *(your goal)*, and discuss progress and challenges with *(the person you'll check in with)* on *(date)*.

(Sign and date your contract, and make any additional notes.)

10. Reward yourself with things that are fun and make you feel good. Make a list of things that that make you feel good that are not food. Let your list include the large and small, free to big-ticket items. What are the ways you are creative? Are you motivated by getting flowers, calling a friend or family member, or getting outside? How do you relax? What would be the biggest gift you could give yourself? When you make your goal, celebrate with a reward. If you don't make your goal but do the work of looking at what made that goal too tough to reach, and how you can make it easier to meet, still take time to celebrate your effort.

Here (pg. 113) is how someone, let's call her Rebecca, might work through this exercise.

REBECCA'S MINDFUL PLAN FOR STARTING HER YOGA PRACTICE

1. Set an intention.

   I feel tired a lot of the time. I know I would probably feel better if I got more physical movement, but I seem to have trouble staying with it. My intention is to find out if a regular yoga practice really does help me manage my blood sugar, and if that will make me feel better. I want to feel more energetic.

2. Identify specific areas for experimentation.

   Physical activity: I don't get much movement.

   Stress: I have a lot of it and know it is impacting my life.

   Food: I love to eat and know I overdo it too often.

3. Set a compassionate goal. What is the experiment?

   I will do yoga at least 3 times each week.

   Now get specific; specify a time period (e.g., week, month, vacation)

   Over the next month

   Specify how often (e.g., daily, once a week)

   Three times per week

   Specify how much (e.g., daily, once a week)

   For at least 10 minutes

   Specify where (e.g., home, restaurant, work)

   Either at home or a local class

   Specify with whom (e.g., family member, friends, co-workers)

   Myself, or with others at the local class

4. Develop affirmations. Write an affirmation that envisions your intention.

   I love my yoga practice: It gives me energy and helps me better manage my blood sugar.

5. Create a visualization.

   I see myself enjoying good health with my family and friends.

6. Develop a plan of action. List the three challenges that you are most likely to encounter in your effort to reach your goal.

   Challenge #1? No time

   Challenge #2? Motivation

   Challenge #3? Forgetting to do it

   (continued on the next page)

("Rebecca's mindful plan" continued from previous page)

What will you do to manage your challenges in order to prevent them from affecting your ability to attain your goal?

To manage challenge #1, I will: Write my practice time into my daily schedule, and make it non-negotiable—a priority.

To manage challenge #2, I will: Give myself a little healthy treat—maybe some yoga clothing or flowers—if I meet my goal. Also, when I know it's time to do my yoga and I don't want to, I will practice mindfulness of thoughts for a few minutes to see if it helps. Then I will practice.

To manage challenge #3, I will: As above, but I'll also place a kind reminder note near my bed to remind me to practice first thing in the morning.

7. **Explore achievability. How confident are you, on a scale of 0–100%, that you can achieve this goal?**

Realistically, I feel like I'm at 60%, but if I say 3x/week on 2 of the next 4 weeks, I'm 80% positive I can do this.

9. **Seal the deal with a contract.**

I will begin working on the following goal and supporting affirmations:

Beginning tomorrow, May 5, I will write three yoga practices into my schedule each week, and check them off when I do them. I will practice at least 3x/week on at least 2 of the next 4 weeks. I will say my affirmation out loud as often as I think of it. I will discuss successes and challenges with my friend Sally, within three days of June 5. When I achieve this excellent month, I will get myself a little yoga gift.

Signed: Rebecca Smith, May 4.

Resistance and setbacks

It seems at times, when you set a nice lofty goal of taking terrific care of yourself, the universe chuckles a bit and says, "Oh yeah? Well, try this one." And zing, a barrier you never even anticipated comes your way. Not meeting your goal is not failure: It is learning. It means that you either have to create an easier goal, or remove barriers that are getting in your way. You are successful if you stay at it and learn from missing the mark. Resistance and strong emotions are a natural part of change. We all feel them. If you let resistance or strong emotions stop you from trying new things or managing your health, and this becomes a pattern, it may prevent you from moving forward. What feelings do you have about your diabetes, or about making a particular change? Why do you think you have those feelings? How do you think your feelings affect your choices? A wise friend, (integrative health practitioner Dharani Burnham) gave me this simple practice for working with emotions. Resistance works the same way.

Working with emotions

Enjoy this simple, mindful practice of working with emotions.

- **Feel it.** How does the emotion or the resistance show up in your body? In your thoughts?

- **Honor it.** Emotions and resistance are messengers. What might have triggered the emotion?

- **Release it.** Thank the emotion or resistance for sharing, and let it go. You might say, "I now release this resistance and will start my practice anyway." Sometimes writing it down on a piece of paper, and burning the paper, is helpful as a ceremony of letting go.

It is highly likely that at some point in the practice you will have some resistance. Remember, resistance is a natural part of change; don't let it derail you. We all feel it—sometimes it seems life can throw obstacles in the way at every turn. Change experts suggest that it takes about 30 days of practice—of working through the resistance and doing it anyway—for a new habit to take hold. So relax, breathe, and know that you don't have to be perfect. No one else is, after all. Keep coming back to it, and give it time to work.

PRACTICE IN LIFE: A 6-WEEK YOGA AND DIABETES PROGRAM

Here is an example of how you might combine your yoga program and the exercises in this chapter for a whole-life yoga and diabetes program.

Week 1: Getting started

- Do step 1 of the Internal Dialogue exercise: noticing your thoughts (pg. 107)
- Complete the Create Your Mindful Lifestyle exercise (pg. 110)
- Do a 10-minute yoga program suited to you at a regular time on most days

Week 2: Internal dialogue

- Complete the Internal Dialogue exercise (pg. 107)
- Practice goals you developed in the Create Your Mindful Lifestyle exercise (pg. 110)
- Do a 10- or 30-minute yoga program at a regular time most days

Week 3: Mindful eating

- Practice awareness of your Internal Dialogue
- Complete the Mindful Eating exercise (pg. 109)
- Practice mindful eating twice or more through the week
- Practice goals from the Create Your Mindful Lifestyle exercise (pg. 110)
- Do a 10- or 30-minute yoga program at a regular time on most days

Week 4: Gratitude

- Complete the Internal Dialogue exercise again, looking for new trends
- Practice Mindful Eating twice or more
- Complete the Gratitude List exercise (pg. 107)
- Review your progress on your goals. If you have not met them, what can you do to make them easier?
- Do a 10- or 30-minute yoga program at a regular time on most days

Week 5: Integration

- Practice Internal Dialogue awareness, Mindful Eating, and/or the Gratitude exercises
- Journaling questions: Take a few moments to write down answers to the following:

  Which practices do you find most helpful?

  Has your overall lifestyle changed? How?

  Do you feel different than when you began? How?

- Do a 10- or 30-minute yoga program at a regular time on most days

Week 6: Complete the spiral

- Practice Internal Dialogue awareness, Mindful Eating, and Gratitude exercises

- Review progress on Create Your Mindful Lifestyle goals or shifts

- With what you have learned from practice and journaling, repeat the Lifestyle exercise, perhaps choosing a new goal or continuing to work on your current goal

- If you have completed this program, you have committed major effort to improving your lifestyle. Celebrate with a healthy indulgence! How can you treat yourself fabulously well in a way that feels good and meets your blood sugar targets?

These steps involve an ongoing process of practicing, noticing how they feel and work, making adjustments, and practicing again. If you find it too difficult to practice regularly, what can you do to make this process easier? Try a shorter practice, or every other day, or even once a week for starters.

The Spiral of Life

If you look closely, spirals are everywhere in nature. The leaves of a dandelion, the limbs of a tree, and ears of corn all unfurl as spirals, as do waves in the ocean. For many, one or two (or more) life issues keep coming around again, perhaps in a different way. As you deepen your practice of yoga, don't be surprised if familiar issues happen in your practice. As one of my wise Kripalu teachers said, yoga activates (brings up things like strong emotions) and yoga integrates (helps us to understand and be at peace with what comes up). Continue with your practice, find a kind and gentle teacher to help guide you, and stretch on.

We wish you a happy and healthy life.

Namaste.

(THIS MEANS THAT THE LIGHT IN ME BOWS TO THE LIGHT IN YOU.)

Glossary

Asana: Sanskrit word meaning "seat." Refers to specific body position used in some postures.

Autonomic dysfunction: This refers to a breakdown in functioning of the autonomic nervous system (ANS). The ANS controls involuntary processes such as the regulation of blood pressure, heart rate, body temperature, and bladder control.

Blood sugar: The amount of glucose (sugar) in the blood. Glucose is the energy currency of the body, but high blood glucose over time is a marker of diabetes.

Central nervous system: Includes the brain and cranial nerves, spinal column, and spinal nerves.

Core: The center of the body from which limbs and neck extend; the trunk or torso. The core includes the thorax and abdomen, and the major organs and muscle groups. Core stability refers to the condition of muscle groups of the trunk that contribute to posture and healthy body functioning.

Diabetic retinopathy: A complication of diabetes that affects the eyes, caused by damage to the blood vessels in the eye.

Engage: To gently contract a muscle or set of muscles. To engage the belly, gently contract the abdominal muscles by drawing the belly button toward the spine. Engage the muscles with slight contraction and lift. You might think of hugging muscles into the bone to engage.

Extension: Movement at a joint that increases the angle of the joint, as in straightening the arm, which extends the elbow. Also, when a body part that moves forward and back moves back, as in when you do a backbend, the spine is extended.

Flexion: Movement at a joint that decreases the angle of the joint. For example, bending your arm at the elbow is flexion. Sitting down in a chair flexes the knee joint.

Gene: The molecular unit of DNA that determines heredity or a genetically determined function.

Glaucoma: A group of eye conditions that result in damage to the optic nerve. High pressure inside the eye sometimes causes the damage.

Heart disease: Cardiovascular disease; a group of conditions involving the circulatory system. Many forms of heart disease are preventable or improved with changes to lifestyle.

High blood pressure: Hypertension. When the pressure inside your blood vessels is high enough to undermine your health, increasing your risk for heart disease and other conditions. Generally the narrower your arteries, the higher your blood pressure.

Hypoglycemia: Low blood sugar. This may be caused by diet, medications, or exercise.

Insulin: A hormone produced by the pancreas that causes cells to absorb glucose from the bloodstream. Important in the metabolism of carbohydrate and fat.

Kumbhaka: Sanskrit word for holding one's breath. It refers to either holding the breath in (internal kumbhaka) or holding the breath out (external kumbhaka).

Lifestyle disease: A medical condition that is the result of poor nutrition and lack of physical activity or other choices like smoking.

Mantra: Sanskrit word for mind-freedom. A practice of meditative repetitive chanting or singing of a word or phrase.

Metabolism: The collection of cellular biochemical reactions and their interplay that sustains life.

Namaste: Sanskrit word used as a form of greeting, parting, and honoring.

Peripheral neuropathy: A result of nerve damage that may cause weakness, numbness, or pain, usually in hands and feet.

Peripheral vascular disease: Refers to any circulatory disease outside the heart and brain. Caused by a buildup of fatty deposits in the artery walls.

Prana: Sanskrit word for energy in its broadest sense. The vital energy that animates the world.

Pranayama: Sanskrit word for breathing and other energy practices of yoga.

Range of motion: The full distance that an object can move when attached to another object. Usually refers to the ability of joints to operate without limitations relative to their optimal function.

Resiliency: The ability to recover or rebound from illness, adversity, or stress.

Root: Press down, as in pressing into the floor as though you could press through the floor into the earth. Anchored.

Sanskrit: An ancient language from India; the language of yoga.

Self-efficacy: An individual's belief in their ability to do something. Confidence in one's ability to pursue behaviors that may help in the management of blood sugars, for example.

Spine: The skeletal structure and the collection of muscles and fascia along the spine.

Supine: Lying down.

Wellness: A state that combines health and happiness. A balance of mind, body, and spirit that results in an overall sense of well-being. Thought to include activities to improve your state of physical, mental, emotional, spiritual, environmental, social, and occupational health.

Yoga: Sanskrit word for union. Thought to refer to union of the mind, body, and spirit. A practice of self-inquiry that includes physical practice and philosophy.

Resources for Further Study

Physical Activity, Diabetes, and Health Resources

AMERICAN DIABETES ASSOCIATION
1701 Beauregard Street
Alexandria, VA 22311
1-800-DIABETES
www.diabetes.org

AMERICAN HEART ASSOCIATION
7272 Greenville Avenue
Dallas, TX 75231
1-800-242-8721
www.heart.org

U.S. CENTERS FOR DISEASE CONTROL
AND PREVENTION
Division of Diabetes Translation
1600 Clifton Road
Atlanta, GA 30333
1-800-232-4636
www.cdc.gov/diabetes

DIVISION OF NUTRITION, PHYSICAL ACTIVITY
AND OBESITY
1600 Clifton Road
Atlanta, GA 30333
1-800-232-4636
www.cdc.gov/nccdphp/dnpa

NATIONAL DIABETES PREVENTION PROGRAM
1600 Clifton Road
Atlanta, GA 30333
1-800-232-6348
www.cdc.gov/diabetes/prevention/

NATIONAL DIABETES EDUCATION PROGRAM
One Diabetes Way
Bethesda, MD 20814-9692
1-800-438-5383
www.yourdiabetesinfo.org/Healthsense

NATIONAL DIABETES INFORMATION
CLEARINGHOUSE
NIDDK, NIH
Building 31, Room 9A06
31 Center Drive, MSC 2560
Bethesda, MD 20893-2560
1-301-496-3583
www.diabetes.niddk.nih.gov

Physical Activity Guidelines for Americans

NATIONAL HEALTH INFORMATION CENTER
PO Box 1133
Washington, DC 20013-1133
1-800-336-4794
www.health.gov/paguidelines/

Yoga Organizations

NATIONAL CENTER FOR COMPLEMENTARY
AND ALTERNATIVE MEDICINE
National Institutes of Health
31 Center Drive, MSC 2182
Bethesda, MD 20892-2182
888-644-6226
www.nccam.nih.gov

YOGA ALLIANCE
1701 Clarendon Boulevard, Suite 100
Arlington, VA 22209
www.yogaalliance.org

INTERNATIONAL ASSOCIATION OF YOGA
THERAPISTS
PO Box 251563
Little Rock, AR 72225
www.iayt.org

KRIPALU CENTER FOR YOGA & HEALTH
PO Box 309
Stockbridge, MA 01262
1-800-741-7353
www.kripalu.org

Yoga, Meditation, and Mindfulness Books and Publications

Yoga Journal's Yoga Basics
Mara Carrico and the editors of Yoga Journal,
Henry Holt (1997)

Yoga and the Quest for the True Self
Stephen Cope, Bantam (2000)

Kripalu Yoga: A Guide to Practice On and Off the Mat
Richard Faulds and the senior teachers at the Kripalu Center for Yoga & Health, Bantam Dell (2006)

Already Home: Stories of a Seeker
Aruni Nan Futuronsky, Cold River Studio (2010)

Touching Peace: Practicing the Art of Mindful Living
Thich Nhat Hahn, Parallax Press (1992)

Light on Yoga
B.K.S. Iyengar, Random House (1966, 1977, 1979)

Every Bite Is Divine: The Balanced Approach to Enjoying Eating, Feeling Healthy and Happy, and Getting to a Weight That's Natural For You
Annie Kay, Life Arts Press (2007)

Meditation for the Love of it
Sally Kempton, Sounds True (2010)

Yoga for Wellness: Healing with the Timeless Teachings of Viniyoga
Gary Kraftsow, Penguin (1999)

Yoga for Transformation: Ancient Teaching and Practices for Healing the Body, Mind and Heart
Gary Kraftsow, Penguin (2002)

The Key Poses of Yoga: Your Guide to Functional Anatomy
Ray Long, Bhanda Yoga Publications (2008)

Yoga: The Iyengar Way
Silva Mehta and Mira Shyam Mehta, Alfred A. Knopf (1990)

Body Stories: A Guide to Experiential Anatomy
Andrea Olsen and Caryn McHose, Station Hill Press (1991)

Yoga: The Spirit and Practice of Moving into Stillness
Erich Schiffmann, Simon & Schuster (1996)

Yoga for Depression: A Compassionate Guide to Relieve Suffering Through Yoga
Amy Weintraub, Harmony Books (2003)

Yoga Journal
2520 55th St, Suite 210
Boulder, CO 80301
415-591-0555
www.yogajournal.com

Index

Note: Page numbers followed by an *f* refer to figures.

brain, 6–7
breath/breathe, 5–6, 10*f*, 12–14, 84, 94–95, 97–100. *See also* breathing practice
breathing in corpse, 86*f*
breathing practice
    alternate nostril breathing, 18, 19*f*, 86*f*, 88*f*, 90*f*–94*f*, 97*f*, 99*f*, 101*f*, 104*f*
    belly breath, 14, 15*f*, 85*f*–86*f*, 89*f*, 92*f*, 94*f*, 101*f*, 103*f*–104*f*
    intentionally holding your breath, 20
    wave-sounding breath, 16, 17*f*, 85*f*, 89*f*, 92*f*–94*f*, 97*f*, 99*f*
bridge, 70, 71*f*, 85*f*, 87*f*–91*f*, 93*f*, 98*f*, 100*f*, 101
Burnham, Dharani, 115

C

calmness, 14, 15*f*
cancer, 5
carbohydrate, 23–24
cardiovascular system, 7
cat and dog, 30, 31*f*, 86*f*, 90*f*, 94*f*
centering posture, 84–85
central nervous system, 6–7, 119
chair, 27
change, 110–112
chest, 58, 59*f*, 60, 61*f*, 70, 71*f*
child, 32, 33*f*, 86*f*, 90*f*–91*f*, 93*f*–94*f*, 97*f*–100*f*
Chödrön, Pema, 83
cholesterol, 3*f*, 8
chronic stress, 6
cleanliness, 10*f*
clinical trial, 3
clothing, 26
cobbler, 66, 67*f*, 92*f*–93*f*, 98*f*, 100*f*, 103*f*–104*f*
cobra, 58, 59*f*, 60, 61*f*, 86*f*, 88*f*, 90*f*, 95*f*–97*f*, 99*f*
comfort, 25–26
compassion, 110–111, 113
compassionate self-observation, 106
complication, 22–23
contentment, 10*f*
contract, 112, 114

core, 42, 46, 48, 72, 74–75, 85, 119
corpse, 21, 80, 81*f*, 85*f*–87*f*, 89*f*–94*f*, 98*f*, 100*f*–101*f*
cortisol, 8
cushion, 26, 28

D

dharana, 10*f*
dhyana, 10*f*
diabetes
    complication, 22–23
    diet-controlled, 22
    gestational, 22, 24, 102
    integrative lifestyle condition, 1–3
    special considerations, 22
    type 1, 22, 24, 102
    type 2, 5, 102
Diabetes Prevention Program (DPP), 2
dialogue, internal, 107
diet, 3*f*, 109–110, 116
diet-controlled diabetes, 22
digestive system, 7, 64, 72, 75*f*, 76, 77*f*
distraction, 13
downward dog, 89*f*–91*f*, 94*f*–97*f*, 99*f*, 100, 102
downward dog against the wall, 56, 57*f*, 102
downward dog on a chair, 56, 57*f*
downward facing dog, 54, 55*f*, 56

E

easy belly breathing. See belly breath
eating, 109–110, 116
elbow, 22
emotion, 6, 13, 115
emotional reasoning, 108
endocrine system, 7
endorphin, 6–7
endurance, 99–100
energy, 6, 13, 72, 73*f*, 74, 75*f*, 90
engage, 119
exenatide, 24

Y